High Flow Nasal Cannula

Annalisa Carlucci · Salvatore M. Maggiore
Editors

High Flow Nasal Cannula

Physiological Effects and Clinical Applications

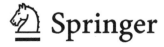 Springer

Editors
Annalisa Carlucci
Department of Medicine
University of Varese and Pulmonary
Rehabilitation Institute
Maugeri
Pavia
Italy

University Department of Innovative
Technologies in Medicine & Dentistry,
Gabriele d'Annunzio University of
Chieti-Pescara
Chieti
Italy

Salvatore M. Maggiore
Clinical Department of Anaesthesiology
and Intensive Care Medicine
SS. Annunziata Hospital
Chieti
Italy

ISBN 978-3-030-42453-4   ISBN 978-3-030-42454-1   (eBook)
https://doi.org/10.1007/978-3-030-42454-1

This Springer imprint is published by the registered company Springer Nature Switzerland AG
The registered company address is: Gewerbestrasse 11, 6330 Cham, Switzerland

Contents

Conventional Oxygen Therapy: Technical and Physiological Issues

1

François Lellouche and Erwan L'Her

"And the LORD God formed man of the dust of the ground, and breathed into his nostrils the breath of life; and man became a living soul" (Genesis 2.7)

"Though pure dephlogisticated air [oxygen] might be very useful as a medicine … as a candle burns out much faster in dephlogisticated air [oxygen] … so we might live out too fast," (Joseph Priestley, Experiments and Observations on Different Kinds of Air, 1775)

1.1 Introduction

High-flow oxygen therapy or high-flow nasal cannula oxygenation is usually defined as administration of gas flow above 15 L/min [1]. Conventional oxygen therapy with low (below 5 L/min) to moderate flows (below or equal to 15 L/min) is one of the most used drugs in hospitals and during prehospital transportation [2–4]. Recently, the studies that demonstrated the twofold increased mortality with hyperoxia in patients with acute respiratory failure [5] and the meta-analyses that found an increased mortality with liberal oxygen use in critically ill patients [6, 7] have revived the debate [8–10]. However, knowledge on oxygen toxicity is heterogeneous for the management of patients with chronic respiratory failure [11] and is extremely poor for other populations such as patients managed for acute myocardial infarction [12]. Recent guidelines are very restrictive concerning the utilization of oxygen in patients at risk to develop hypercapnia such as COPD patients [13] but beyond these patients for all acutely ill patients admitted in hospital [14].

F. Lellouche (✉)
Centre de Recherche de l'Institut Universitaire de Cardiologie et de Pneumologie de Québec, Québec, QC, Canada
e-mail: francois.lellouche@criucpq.ulaval.ca

E. L'Her
CHU La Cavale Blanche, Brest, France

© Springer Nature Switzerland AG 2021
A. Carlucci, S. M. Maggiore (eds.), *High Flow Nasal Cannula*,
https://doi.org/10.1007/978-3-030-42454-1_1

Oxygen is considered as one of the most important chemical elements necessary to the metabolism and energy production for all living beings [15]. Next to the vital need of oxygen known by general public and health practitioners, the flip side of the oxygen and dangers associated with this gas should also be known. Deleterious effects of excessive oxygen delivery have long been described, particularly in patients with chronic obstructive pulmonary disease (COPD) [16] and in neonates [17, 18] for more than half a century. There is also a growing evidence of the systemic toxicity of oxygen due to cellular damages and vascular toxicity in many patients (coronary artery disease, stroke, critically ill patients). Because of the dangers associated with hypoxemia as well as those related to hyperoxemia, precise adjustment and restrictive use of oxygen are now recommended [13, 14]. Yet, despite being one of the most commonly administered treatments in the hospital, the goal of precise adjustment seems difficult to achieve so far [3, 4, 19, 20]. We will review the physiological effects of oxygen and the risks associated with hypoxemia and those associated with hyperoxia and hyperoxemia.

The methods to deliver oxygen have not changed a lot over the last century [21]. We will review the different devices used to deliver oxygen and the recommended monitoring of this therapy. We will also review the innovative methods that have recently been developed to accurately titrate oxygen, the automated oxygen delivery systems [22–26].

1.2 Conventional Oxygen Therapy

1.2.1 Historical Overview of Oxygen Discovery and Utilization

Dioxygen (O_2) was discovered at the end of the eighteenth century by Carl Schiele, Joseph Priestley, and Antoine Lavoisier [27] (Fig. 1.1). More recently, the importance of the work of Michael Sendivogius (1566–1636) was underlined in the path of the discovery of oxygen [28]. More than 150 years before the well-known trio reputed for oxygen discovery, this Polish alchemist could already produce "the food of life" later called oxygen by heating saltpetre (potassium nitrate) [28]. This gas has long been considered as a magical and almost holy gas, initially called the "breath of life" in the Bible, "elixir of life," "food of life," "vital air," and "dephlogisticated air" before Lavoisier named it *oxy-gen* in 1777, meaning acid generator [29, 30]. Both Priestley and Lavoisier described the major role of oxygen to sustain life and they also described the potential lung toxicity, only few years after initial discoveries [29, 31]. First clinical utilization of oxygen in 1783 is attributed to Caillens, a French physician [32]. After Beddoes and Watt's work [33], oxygen and other medical gases were studied and administered to patients at a larger scale at the Pneumatic Institution (1798–1802), Bristol, England. Initial results were heterogeneous due to very wide initial indications for oxygen administration (consumption-pulmonary tuberculosis, king's evil-cervical tuberculosis, asthma, dropsy, palsy …) [34, 35], and possibly due to impurities in the initial oxygen production [36]. Another major obstacle to a large utilization was the difficulties related to oxygen

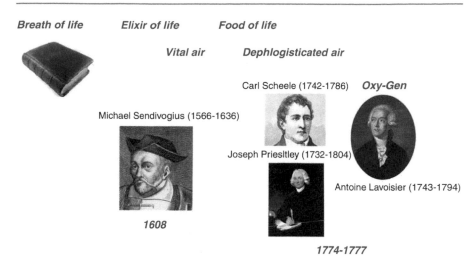

Fig. 1.1 The discovery of oxygen, from the "breath of life" in the Bible to the Oxy/Gen. During centuries, before it was named "oxygen" by Lavoisier, this gas was considered like a magical gas, and it was soon understood that it was vital for all living beings. However, immediately after its discovery, the potential toxicity was suspected by Priestley and Lavoisier

production, transportation, and administration. Sometimes used pure or in combination with nitrous oxide, the first cylinders for storing oxygen were developed in the second half of the century, in 1868 [34]. Physiologic role of oxygen and modes of administration were extensively studied in the twentieth century and several researchers such as John Scott Haldane (1860–1936) (who described the effects of hypoxia during the Pikes Peak expedition [37, 38] and the "Haldane effect" [39]), his son John Burdon Sanderson Haldane (1892–1964) (who described the neurological effects of hyperoxia in hyperbaric conditions [40, 41]), and Alvan Leroy Barach (1895–1977) [42] provided a scientific rationale to the medical use of oxygen and improvement in the technical aspect for oxygen administration.

The ways to administer oxygen have changed a lot since its discovery, which may explain the slowness to demonstrate the clinical beneficial effects. Oxygen was initially delivered intermittently due to the fear of lung toxicity. The recommended doses were small, typical therapy being "four gallons [approximately 15 liters] morning and evening, usually delivered in few minutes from a bucket towards the face of the patient" [35]. The intermittent use as well as the device to deliver oxygen may explain in part the initial disappointing results. The first description of continuous use of oxygen was made by Blodgett in 1890 [43]. At the beginning of the twentieth century, Haldane also recommended the continuous delivery of oxygen to treat injuries caused by chlorine gas during the First World War [44, 45]. Haldane said, "intermittent oxygen therapy is like bringing a drowning man to the surface of the water—occasionally." In spite of the benefits of continuous administration of oxygen, there was still reluctance on the part of the medical profession to administer oxygen continuously due to the fear of oxygen toxicity. Oxygen was still mainly provided intermittently, until Campbell recommendations in 1960 [46]. Finally, in

1962 Massaro et al. demonstrated that intermittent administration of oxygen … had only intermittent effects on oxygenation and that oxygen could lead to increased CO_2 retention in some patients [47]. In 1973, 34% of the clinicians still provided intermittent oxygen to patients, either often (11%) or rarely (23%) [48]. Currently, almost all physicians use oxygen continuously but this has not always been the standard, and the pendulum is still swinging: after a phase of liberal use, new studies and recommendations are moving towards a more restrictive use and a strict adjustment [6, 13, 14]. The recent recommendations are a turning point in the story of oxygen. The new statement is that healthcare practitioners should be worried about hyperoxemia such as they are with hypoxemia: a turning point … or a return to the initial mitigated feelings of Lavoisier and Priestley for oxygen, a vital and toxic gas!

1.2.2   Updated Recommendations for Oxygen Utilization

The first goal of oxygen therapy is still to treat hypoxemia in acutely ill patients (mainly during respiratory or cardiac failure) [13, 14]. The other objective which is recommended but frequently disregarded is to avoid hyperox(em)ia [13, 14]. First recommendations to deliver oxygen have been published by Campbell in 1960. He recommended continuous delivery, low FiO_2 administration (24–35%), and reduction of expiratory gas rebreathing to avoid CO_2 accumulation [46]. These recommendations focused on COPD patients. Since initial recommendations, others are regularly issued from different national or international societies [13, 49, 50]. Interestingly, in most guidelines, the focus was only on the minimum level of oxygenation to deliver (minimum SpO_2) until recently. Maximum SpO_2 values were only recommended for COPD patients and in neonate populations [51], as underlined by Semienuk et al. [14]. A maximum SpO_2 was first recommended by the Thoracic Society of Australia and New Zealand for other categories of patients, and these recommendations were called "swimming between the flags" [50]. The most recent recommendations provide a target SpO_2 range with a minimum and a maximum SpO_2 value [13, 14]. This may seem like a minor change to the protocols, while it actually changes the whole challenge of management and monitoring for the clinicians.

The main recommendations for oxygen therapy in critically ill patients may be summarized as follows (Fig. 1.2):

1. Use oxygen only to treat hypoxemia and neither to treat breathlessness nor thoracic pain.
2. Use a restrictive rather than a liberal strategy to deliver oxygen.
3. SpO_2 target should be between 88 and 92% in patients at risk of hypercapnia (not only for COPD patients) which is quite consistent in the different guidelines (while relying on few data).
4. For other populations, there is a discrepancy in recommendations. Minimal SpO_2 targets vary from 90% to 94% and maximal SpO_2 targets vary from 94% to 98% [13, 14, 50]. The most recent recommendations, which are derived from the meta-analyses comparing liberal and conservative oxygen administration, are

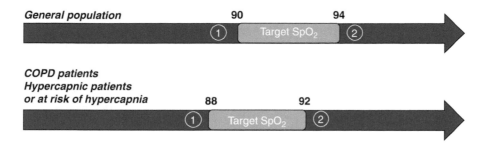

Fig. 1.2 Recommendations for oxygenation targets in the general population [14] and in patients with hypercapnia or at risk of hypercapnia (COPD, severe obesity …) [13]. SpO_2 values below OR above the SpO_2 target should be considered dangerous for the patients. ① represents the SpO_2 values for which oxygen supplementation should be initiated. ② represents the SpO_2 values for which the oxygen supplementation should be stopped or minimized to attain the SpO_2 target

the most radical for a restrictive use and strongly recommend to stop oxygen if SpO_2 is above 96% and not to start oxygen if SpO_2 is equal to or above 93% [14]. The recommended SpO_2 target is 90–94%.

5. SpO_2 should be closely monitored and even continuously monitored for most severe patients, and arterial blood gases should only be used in case of potential hypercapnia or metabolic disorders.
6. NEWS or equivalent scoring system should be monitored in patients receiving oxygen to allow an early detection of clinical worsening [13].
7. Oxygen supplementation improves oxygenation, but the underlying cause of hypoxemia must be treated.

The knowledge transfer concerning oxygen therapy is among the worst example. Indeed, it seems difficult to comply with recommendations and guidelines for oxygen prescription and delivery existing for more than 50 years [19, 52–54]. This may be explained by several obstacles including the belief that oxygen cannot be harmful, despite recent evidence demonstrating oxygen toxicity even in the general population [6]. However, even in COPD patients for which hypercapnia induced by hyperoxemia was described 70 years ago, prescription is still frequently not adequate [19]. In most situations, too much oxygen is provided to patients and oxygen toxicity is frequently overlooked. We will underline below the impact of oxygen therapy complications, with both hypoxemia and hyperoxemia being life threatening.

1.3 Physiological Effects of Oxygen and Toxicity

1.3.1 Physiological Role of Oxygen and Cellular Toxicity

Dioxygen (O_2) is used in mitochondria for aerobic cellular respiration leading to the production of adenosine triphosphate (ATP) via oxidative phosphorylation which is the main way to store energy and powers most cellular reactions in eukaryotes [55].

CO_2 and H_2O are produced as well as energy stored in the form of ATP during the process. The aerobic respiration is the following simplified reaction: $C_6H_{12}O_6 + 6$ $O_2 \rightarrow 6\,CO_2 + 6\,H_2O + 2880$ kJ/mol. Aerobic pathway is considered at least 15 times more efficient to produce ATP: anaerobic produces only 2-molecule ATP per 1-molecule glucose while 30- to 38-molecule ATP can be produced with 1-molecule glucose through aerobic respiration [56]. Electron transport chains in the mitochondria are major sites of electron leakage. Oxygen serves as an effective electron acceptor (oxidizing agent), generating reactive oxygen species (ROS), also called free radicals, such as superoxide ion (O_2-), hydrogen peroxide (H_2O_2), and the most reactive one hydroxyl radical (OH-) [57]. The toxicity of these free radicals relies on their different reactivity and lifetime. Hydrogen peroxide (H_2O_2) is less reactive with a half-life of few minutes while hydroxyl radical (OH-) is the most reactive and immediately removes electrons from any molecule in its path and thus propagates a chain reaction, which explains its extremely short lifetime estimated in nanoseconds [58, 59]. The combination of different free radicals and especially the hydrogen peroxide in the presence of Fe2+ ions can produce the very highly reactive and damaging hydroxyl radical (OH-) (Fenton reaction) [60]. However, hydrogen peroxide (H_2O_2) may also be damaging to DNA since its lower reactivity provides enough time for the molecule to travel into the nucleus of the cell, subsequently reacting with macromolecules such as DNA.

In a biological context, ROS not only are toxic molecules and but also have important roles in cell signaling, homeostasis, and immune system with direct toxicity against bacteria and other pathogens [57, 61, 62]. Accurate regulation rather than elimination of ROS is consequently the objective of the protection mechanisms.

With the view of an evolution biochemist who described all the mechanisms to protect living organisms from ROS since almost 4 billion years, we can state that "our whole body is an antioxidant machine" with the aim not to eliminate but to regulate the level of oxygen and ROS at the cellular level [63]. There are several mechanisms to protect cells and to regulate oxygen and ROS concentrations. Several organisms produce mucus layers to reduce oxygen diffusion and oxygen scavengers (leghemoglobin in plants and hemoglobin in animals) and allow storage, transport, and progressive delivery of oxygen to tissues to avoid high oxygen concentrations at cellular levels. Oxygen partial pressure in the ambient air is usually around 160 mmHg (21% of a normobaric atmosphere, 760 mmHg) and enters the pulmonary capillaries at around 100 mmHg with the main oxygen reservoir in hemoglobin. At the other extremity of the oxygen cascade, oxygen pressure in cells is variable and below 10 mmHg in the mitochondria [64]. Oxygen is continuously consumed in the respiratory chain to produce energy, increasing the gradient and the "call of oxygen." Enzymatic (catalase, superoxide dismutase, glutathione peroxidase) and nonenzymatic antioxidants (vitamins A, C, and E, carotenoids …) are also precisely regulating the intracellular concentrations of ROS. These mechanisms limit the dangerously high concentrations of free radicals leading to potential lesions of mitochondrial and cell membranes through lipid peroxidation, and DNA strand breaks and other intracellular macromolecule hits and enzyme inhibitions [65]. In the case of excessive damages, cellular apoptosis may occur. However, despite antioxidant mechanisms, due to environmental stress (e.g., UV or heat exposure), or biological stress (hypoxemia, hyperoxemia, sepsis, ischemia), the ROS levels can increase dramatically. This may result in significant damage to cell structures. The disequilibrium between antioxidants and oxidants is known as oxidative stress, which is promoted during hyperoxia and hyperoxemia [66].

1.3.2 Oxygen Is a Dangerous Gas!

Oxygen is one of the most dangerous gases on the planet. Severinghaus and Astrup described oxygen with humor as follows: "Oxygen is the first atmospheric pollutant. Oxygen is toxic. It rusts a person in a century or less. With oxygen came the danger of fire. If introduced today, this gas might have difficulty getting approved by the Food and Drug Administration" [67]. Indeed, all living species on earth have had to protect themselves against oxygen, from the very beginning of life, more than 3.5 billion years ago. First prokaryotes and eukaryotes were bioengineered with antioxidants, even when oxygen concentration in the air was very low (below 1%) [68]. Almost 3.8 billion years ago, the LUCA (last universal cellular ancestor), ancestor of Eukarya, Bacteria, and Archaea, was equipped with several mechanisms to protect from oxygen (mucus layer, antioxidants such as catalase and superoxide dismutase) [68–71]. These defenses are probably inherent to common mechanisms of toxicity shared by oxygen and X-ray [72]. In both situations, reactive oxygen species (ROS) are produced, from H_2O with X-ray or from oxygen degradation during oxygen metabolism (Fig. 1.3). Before increasing levels of oxygen in the atmosphere (after the great oxidation event that appeared with

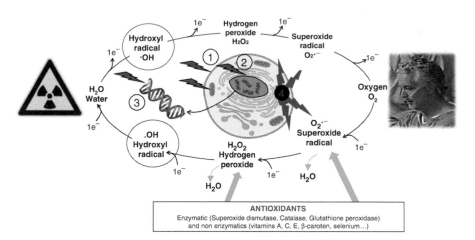

Fig. 1.3 Common mechanisms of toxicity are shared by oxygen and radioactivity [72]. In both situations, reactive oxygen species (ROS) are produced leading to membrane cell damage ①, intracellular membrane damages ②, DNA damage ③, and apoptosis ④. The concentration of the most reactive (hydroxyl radical) is higher with radioactivity. Antioxidant mechanisms reduce the concentration of ROS and limit the toxicity

photosynthesis 2.5 billion years ago), first living cells were exposed to X-rays and acquired these antioxidant mechanisms [63]. Considering this subtle equilibrium, and the different antioxidant defenses acquired during the last 4 billion years, oxygen should not be considered only as a vital gas, but also as a toxic gas. Noteworthy, in normal environments, current *Homo sapiens* only experience normoxia (breathing air with 21% oxygen) or hypoxia in altitude. Hyperoxia (high oxygen intakes) and hyperoxemia (high oxygen concentration in blood) may only be encountered in hospitals or in oxygen bars!

1.3.3   Risks Associated with Hypoxemia

It is not difficult to convince clinicians (and probably anyone crossed in the street, as oxygen is very popular) that the lack of oxygen may be dangerous and life threatening. Several mechanisms of hypoxemia are well described and comprise hypoxia (mainly when living in altitude [73] or induced hypoxemia in laboratory [24, 74]), reduced diffusion (interstitial lung diseases), hypoventilation (drug overdoses, neurological diseases), ventilation/perfusion mismatch (COPD, asthma, pulmonary embolism), intrapulmonary shunt (cardiogenic pulmonary edema, pneumonia, pulmonary embolism), intracardiac shunt, and shock state (cardiogenic, hypovolemic …). Causes of tissue hypoxia are also well described, mainly in the case of sepsis (failure in peripheral oxygen extraction) and several intoxications (CO, cyanide intoxication …). Acute hypoxemia leads to tachycardia (to increase cardiac output and oxygen transport to tissues) [75], increased minute ventilation (to increase oxygen intake) [76, 77], systemic arterial vasodilatation [78, 79], pulmonary vasoconstriction [80], increased tissue extraction of oxygen, and other mechanisms that increase oxygen delivery to tissues (such as right shift of the hemoglobin saturation curve). Other physiological compensations exist to counterbalance hypoxemia in the case of subacute or chronic hypoxia (in populations living in altitude) or chronic hypoxemia (mainly in cardiorespiratory diseases), primarily the polycythemia.

When the protection mechanisms are overwhelmed, tissue hypoxia may occur, with risks of cardiac ischemia (especially due to associated tachycardia), cardiac arrhythmia [81, 82], hepatic ischemia, cerebral ischemia, and cellular anaerobic respiration leading to increased lactate production [83].

To correct hypoxemia, oxygen must be administered urgently, but this is only a supportive therapy and etiological treatment must be adequately provided. The most recent recommendations are to deliver oxygen to maintain SpO_2 above 88% in patients at risk of hypercapnia and 90% in other patients [14]. Oxygen supplementation should be initiated only if SpO_2 is below 93% in the general population (Fig. 1.2).

1.3.4 Risks Associated with Hyperoxia: Oxygen Toxicity (Fig. 1.4)

It is less intuitive to endorse that oxygen may be toxic and increases mortality [5–7, 84]. Oxygen toxicity is low-grade toxicity or hidden from view in most circumstances which may explain that it is neglected. However, the deleterious effects of oxygen have been described very early after oxygen discovery by Lavoisier and Priestley [29, 31] and compelling demonstrations are now available that hyperoxia may lead to increased mortality [5–7, 84, 85]. There have been more than 7000 publications on hyperoxia in the last 70 years on "PubMed," with an exponential increase after the introduction of pulse oximetry in the clinical practice in the early 1980s. Most publications are descriptions of physiological mechanisms of toxicity [65] but in the last 10 years, several randomized clinical trials have described more accurately this toxicity and allowed to better figure out the real impact of hyperoxemia in different populations. First demonstrations of increased risk of liberal use of oxygen were provided in 2010 by Austin et al. [5]. The authors evaluated

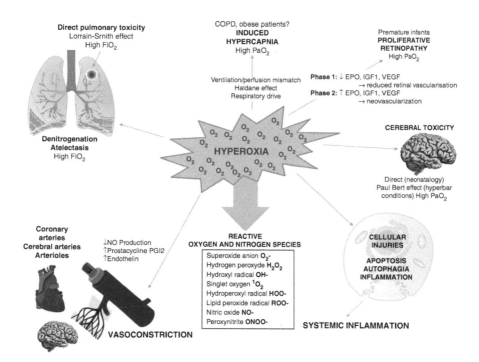

Fig. 1.4 Systemic toxicity of oxygen. Oxygen toxicity involves several organs. The cellular as well as vascular toxicity makes the toxicity of oxygen systemic. This may explain the deleterious effects of oxygen leading to increased mortality when used liberally [6]

the impact of oxygen flow rate delivered to patients managed in ambulances for acute respiratory distress. Mortality was significantly lower in patients receiving titrated oxygen (targeting a SpO_2 of 88–92%) rather than high-concentration oxygen (8–10 L/min of oxygen flow rate): 9% vs. 4%, $p = 0.02$; relative risk, 0.42; and 95% confidence interval 0.20–0.89. In the subgroup of patients with confirmed chronic obstructive pulmonary disease ($n = 214$) mortality was reduced even further (9% vs. 2%, $p = 0.04$; 0.22, 0.05–0.91). This effect was shown despite a mean exposure of only 47 min [5]. This study has limitations, including a low compliance to protocols, especially in the targeted oxygen arm (only 41% compliance rate). A recently published randomized controlled trial conducted in critically ill mechanically ventilated patients further revived the interest in this often-minimized question of oxygen toxicity. This study conducted in 434 mechanically ventilated patients showed a clear increase in mortality (20.2% vs. 11.6%, $p = 0.01$) in patients in the hyperoxic group (SpO_2 target of 97–100%) in comparison with normoxic patients (target SpO_2 94–98%) [7]. Recent reports described an impressive U-shaped curve of the impact of mean PaO_2 in critically ill patients [84]. Similarly, short-term exposure to hyperoxemia (median of 5.4 h) in patients intubated at the emergency department was associated with increased mortality [86].

Finally, the meta-analysis recently published by Chu et al. concluded that liberal oxygen use increased mortality in comparison with restrictive oxygen use in different populations of critically ill patients [6].

1.3.4.1 Direct Oxygen Lung Toxicity

Few years after oxygen discovery, Lavoisier described oxygen toxicity and pneumonitis with inflammation of the lungs in animals exposed to pure oxygen, dying from acute respiratory distress after a few days [29]. These initial descriptions were confirmed and extensively described by Lorrain Smith in animals [87]. He described the impact of both oxygen concentration and duration of exposure, known as "Lorrain Smith" effect. These early demonstrations of oxygen toxicity were confirmed by numerous animal studies, reviewed by Clark and Lambertsen [88]. It is now considered that prolonged utilization of high FiO_2 must be avoided to avoid both hypercapnia-induced, direct lung toxicity and denitrogenation atelectasis [89].

1.3.4.2 Importance of Accurate Titration of Oxygen Flow Rates in COPD Patients

Hypoxemia is frequently encountered in severe COPD and is responsible for various severe complications [90]. In addition to the impact of desaturations on pulmonary arterial pressure [91], there are also well-known cardiac effects (myocardial ischemia, tachycardia …) [81, 82].

The risks of hypoxemia are easy to understand and are intuitive, but the risks associated with hyperoxia, and in particular induced hypercapnia, are still neglected [8]. This complication has been known for a long time and was initially suspected by Barach in 1931 [92] and then reported by several authors in 1949 [16, 93, 94]. This effect of oxygen is linked to several mechanisms, such as a decrease in hypoxemic stimulation of the respiratory centers (decrease in minute ventilation [94, 95]), a modification of the ventilation/perfusion ratios [96], or a Haldane effect (reduced affinity of hemoglobin for CO_2 in case of hyperoxia [39]), but the respective role of these mechanisms has long been discussed [96–99]. Campbell published in 1960 and 1967 the first recommendations to adjust the oxygen supply to the minimum [46, 100]. Similar recommendations have since been recently published [13] based on several studies demonstrating that hyperoxemia could induce hypercapnia in some COPD patients [96–99, 101]. Unfortunately, it is well documented that these recommendations are not followed [3, 19] and that patients receive too much oxygen [102] or under certain circumstances not enough [103–105]. The recent demonstration of the risk of excess mortality due to over-oxygenation during the short period of prehospital transport [5] has rekindled the debate [8].

This complication of oxygen therapy seems clinically relevant especially in the context of acute exacerbations [5, 96, 106]. In stable COPD patients, the impact of hyperoxemia on $PaCO_2$ seems to be lower [96, 99]. However, despite the known risks of hypercapnia associated with hyper-oxygenation, many patients treated for exacerbation receive excessive oxygen flow rate [102, 106, 107]. It has recently been shown that high oxygen flow increases mortality in patients managed in ambulances for acute respiratory failure in comparison with oxygen administered to target SpO_2 between 88 and 92% [5]. Likewise, in this population, the negative impact of respiratory acidosis on the prognosis has been well demonstrated, as well as the importance of controlling oxygenation [106–108].

Given the workload especially in emergency situations and the underestimation of the problem, recommendations [13] to limit oxygen flow in COPD are poorly followed [3, 8, 19, 20].

Inhaled aerosols may be used to deliver molecules (especially bronchodilators), which may require gas flows above 6 L/min with pneumatic devices. Consequently, the recommended driving gas is the air to avoid induced hypercapnia, especially in COPD patients [5, 8, 13]. Gunawardena et al. evaluated the driving gas for nebulization and compared oxygen with air in patients with COPD or airway obstruction. This study showed that $PaCO_2$ increased by 7.7 mmHg after nebulization with oxygen as driving gas in patients with baseline hypercapnia. $PaCO_2$ did not increase when air was the driving gas, and in patients without hypercapnia at baseline. Noteworthy, the $PaCO_2$ returned to baseline after 20 min [109]. These data have been recently confirmed in several studies [110, 111]. Another solution if air is not available as driving gas is to perform the nebulization with ultrasonic aerosols which do not require driving gas [112]. In the study of Austin et al. demonstrating a reduced mortality with restrictive use of oxygen during the prehospital transportation in ambulances, nebulizations were delivered with compressed air in the restrictive group [5]. However, this may be difficult to implement in the real-life setting.

1.3.4.3 Vascular Risks Associated with Hyperoxia Are Now Well Demonstrated

There is a significant vascular risk associated with hyperoxemia. It has now been well demonstrated that hyperoxemia notably causes vasoconstriction mediated by a decrease in nitric oxide at the endothelium level [113]. The free radicals (superoxide ions O_2-, peroxide H_2O_2, hydroxyl radical $OH-$ ...) are very reactive and result in a cascade of reactions leading to the reduction of NO concentrations, and consequently to coronary, cerebral, and microvascular vasoconstriction; myocardial dysfunction; and inflammatory response [113]. This effect appears to be rapid, since exposure to 15 min of hyperoxemia in patients with stable coronary artery disease results in a 30% reduction in coronary blood flow and an increase in coronary heart resistance of 30% [114]. In 1959, West and Guzman demonstrated this effect in dogs exposed for 5 min to 100% oxygen [79]. In addition to numerous physiological data [115], clinical studies are now available that better evaluate the clinical impact of hyperoxemia in this population. Recently, Stub et al. have demonstrated in a randomized trial involving 441 patients in the acute phase of myocardial infarction that routine administration of oxygen (at 8 L/min or about 60% FiO_2) was detrimental compared to oxygen administration in case of desaturation below 94% SpO_2 (this situation involved only 8% of patients in this arm) [116]. In the group receiving liberal oxygen, the cardiac enzymes were significantly higher, and the recurrence of infarction was increased, as well as arrhythmia. In 32% of included patients, myocardial MRI was performed 6 months after the initial episode and showed a greater size of the infarct in the oxygen-treated group (20.3 vs. 13.1 g, $p = 0.04$) [116]. A post hoc analysis of a randomized controlled trial involving 1386 patients undergoing abdominal surgery also demonstrated the increased risk of postoperative myocardial infarction with liberal oxygen administration [117]. The main objective of the PROXI trial was to evaluate the impact of perioperative FiO_2 (during surgery and 2 h after) on infections at the surgical site, comparing 30 and 80% of FiO_2 [118]. In the hyperoxic group, the risk of postoperative myocardial infarction was significantly increased: 2.2% vs. 0.9%, 80% vs. 30% FiO_2, HR 2.86 (95% CI 1.10–7.44), as well as several secondary outcomes such as any heart disease or death (HR 1.24 95% CI 1.06–1.45) [117]. Very recently, Hofmann et al. demonstrated in a randomized controlled study that included 6629 patients at the acute phase of myocardial infarction that routine oxygen administration (at 6 L/min or approximately 45% FiO_2) did not reduce mortality compared with administration only in case of desaturation [119]. This demonstrates the uselessness of the routine and liberal administration of oxygen in these patients. As previously noticed, oxygen toxicity seems to be dose dependent [120], since no toxicity was noted with FiO_2 equivalent to 45% [119], while at or above 60%, there seems to exist a coronary and myocardial toxicity [115–117, 121, 122]. In addition, systematic oxygen administration has been proposed to reduce thoracic pain. Recently, Sparv et al. did not find any analgesic effect of routine oxygen as compared with ambient air during myocardial infarction [123]. High-dose oxygen should not be *systematically* administered in the case of myocardial infarction or thoracic pain as it has been done for a long time [10]. Oxygen has long been one of the bases for the management of myocardial infarction at the acute phase. MONA (morphine, oxygen, nitrogen, aspirin) [124] guidelines now tend to recommend oxygen therapy only in patients with acute coronary disease associated with hypoxemia [125]. In the most recent guidelines, it is recommended not to begin oxygen supplementation if SpO_2 is above or equal to 90% [14].

1.3.4.4 Neurological Toxicity

Direct neurological toxicity of oxygen in hyperbaric conditions leading to convulsions has been initially described by Paul Bert in 1878 in the context of hyperbaric hyperoxia in animals [126]. JBS Haldane (the son) reproduced the experiments on himself and described thresholds of oxygen on epilepsy in hyperbaric conditions. He and his collaborator had seizure at approximately the pressure of seven atmospheres layer within 5 min [41, 127]. Haldane also described during these experiments a peripheral neuropathy similar to that found in the Hyper 2S study in patients with septic shock comparing normoxia and 100% FiO_2 for 24 h in critically ill patients [128]. Indeed polyneuropathy was found in 6% vs. 11% in the hyperoxia group ($p = 0.06$) of the patients in the study of Asfar et al. comparing 24 h of pure oxygen administration (100%) to FiO_2 titrated to maintain 88–95% FiO_2 [128]. This study was stopped prematurely because adverse events were significantly more frequent with pure oxygen (including atelectasis, polyneuropathy, renal failure …). In addition to the direct cerebral toxicity mainly in hyperbaric conditions, a 20–30% reduction in cerebral blood flow was found when high FiO_2 was used [129, 130].

1.3.4.5 Oxygen Toxicity in Perioperative and Critical Care Patients

A recently published randomized controlled trial revived interest in this often-minimized question of critical care oxygen toxicity. This study in 434 mechanically ventilated patients demonstrated an increase in mortality (20.2% vs. 11.6%, RR (95% CI): 0.086 (0.017–0.150), $p = 0.01$) in the hyperoxic group (SpO_2 target of 97–100%) in comparison with the normoxic group (SpO_2 target of 94–98%) [7]. Despite limitations discussed in the editorial, this study pointed out that in the acutely ill patients, oxygen should be titrated to target normoxemia and avoid hyperoxemia [131].

There are several types of toxicities in mechanically ventilated patients that may explain these results: impact of hyperoxia (high FiO_2) and effects of "hyperoxemia" (high PaO_2) (Fig. 1.4) [6, 132, 133]. These data may in part be transposed to nasal high-flow therapy or moderate oxygen flow administration.

Among the effects of *hyperoxia*, two types of effects should be considered separately: direct lung toxicity [89] and denitrogenation derecruitment [134]. On the one hand a direct "toxicity" of oxygen exists, initially described in animal studies by Lavoisier [29], then by Lorrain Smith in 1899 [87] and Clark and Lambertsen reviewed more than 100 animal and human studies [88]. This review demonstrated that prolonged exposure and intensity of hyperoxia had an impact on multiple structural components of the lungs. However, toxicity is heterogeneous among species. For example, amphibians may survive indefinitely when exposed to 100% oxygen at atmospheric pressures, while the rat or mouse usually dies after few days' exposure to the same concentration of oxygen [88]. In humans, the clinical importance of lung toxicity related to oxygen remains controversial [89], but it is generally accepted that prolonged administration of FiO_2 above 60% should be avoided, when possible. The other type of lung toxicity with high FiO_2 is explained by denitrogenation atelectasis described in patients under general anesthesia [134–136] and during the ARDS [137]. In the study conducted by Ihnken et al., the impact of oxygenation during coronary artery bypass grafting was evaluated in a randomized controlled study in 40 patients: 20 patients in the hyperoxia group (mean PaO_2 = 419 mmHg) and 20 patients in a "normoxia" group (mean PaO_2 = 142 mmHg) [121]. In addition to the impact on ischemia-reperfusion injuries, in oxidative myocardial damage leading to increased cardiac enzymes in the hyperoxic group, the impact on lung volumes was compelling. Koksal et al. showed similar data with increased oxidative stress and reduced lung volumes in the hyperoxia group in patients managed during abdominal surgery with 80 vs. 40% FiO_2 [138].

Finally, there is a toxicity related to "hyperoxemia" corresponding to high levels of PaO_2 (PaO_2 > 100 mmHg), which is often called inadequately hyperoxia. This systemic toxicity is related to various mechanisms: the production of ROS (free radicals) responsible for "oxidative stress," the vascular toxicity (arterial and arteriolar vasoconstriction), the cellular toxicity, and the induced inflammation (Fig. 1.4). In an observational cohort study including 14,441 mechanically ventilated patients and 295,079 arterial blood gas analyses, Helmerhorst et al. showed that the mean PaO_2 during ICU stay had a strong relationship with mortality [84]. The U-shape relationship demonstrated an increased mortality with hypoxemia as well as hyperoxemia. This U-shape relationship between PaO_2 and mortality has been underlined in several papers [84, 133, 139–141]. In Van der Boom et al.'s study, two US databases were analyzed including more than 35,000 ICU patients with hourly physiological data [141]. In addition to the U-shape relationship between SpO_2 and mortality, the authors found that the percentage of time patients were within an optimal range of SpO_2 was associated with a significant decrease in hospital mortality. When comparing the mortality with 80% vs. 40% of the measurements within the optimal range of oxygenation, the ORs were 0.42 [95% CI, 0.40–0.43] for one database and 0.53 [95% CI, 0.50–0.55] for the other database [141].

A systematic review and meta-analysis demonstrated benefits of normoxemia in comparison with hypoxemia and hyperoxemia in several acutely ill populations (head trauma and stroke, post-cardiac arrest, and mechanical ventilation) [132]. A meta-analysis including 25 randomized controlled trials and 16,037 patients with sepsis, critical illness, stroke, trauma, myocardial infarction, cardiac arrest, and emergency surgery has been recently published in The Lancet journal [6]. This study showed in this population that liberal oxygen therapy increases mortality without improving other patient-important outcomes and concluded that supplemental oxygen with oxygenation above an SpO_2 range of 94–96% may be detrimental to patients [6, 9]. This study and others published previously are the basis of the most recent recommendations to avoid oxygen therapy if SpO_2 is equal or above 93% and to stop oxygen if SpO_2 is above 96% in patients managed for acute care in hospitals [14].

Two large and recently published RCTs have compared two oxygen therapy strategies and did not find differences between study arms [142, 143]. The ICU-ROX study conducted in Australia and New Zealand compared conservative oxygen therapy and usual oxygen therapy in 1000 adults undergoing mechanical ventilation [142]. There was no differences in ventilator-free days and other outcomes. In both study arms, the time-weighted mean daily PaO_2 after inclusion was below 100 mmHg, which suggests that two conservative strategies were compared and may explain the absence of difference found between groups [142]. The inclusions in the study started after the implementation of the Thoracic Society of Australia and New Zealand oxygen guidelines, "swimming between the flags" which may explain that the usual oxygen strategy was a conservative strategy [50, 142]. A very recent RCT has compared two oxygenation targets in 2928 patients with acute hypoxemic respiratory failure [143]. PaO_2 targets were 60 mmHg in the "lower oxygenation" arm and 90 mmHg in the "higher oxygenation" arm. Again, median values of daily PaO_2 were below 100 mmHg in both study arms and no differences in outcome could be detected [143]. Unfortunately, even if patients enrolled in the usual oxygen therapy in the ROX-ICU study had quite low mean PaO_2, this groups was counted in the "higher oxygenation" group in a meta-analysis, which induces a major bias in the analyses and explains the absence of difference between "higher" and "lower" oxygenation strategies [144].

1.3.4.6 Oxygen Toxicity in Premature Infants

There is well-documented oxygen toxicity in premature infants, particularly for the retina and brain [145, 146]. Retinopathy of prematurity "Terry syndrome" associated with hyperoxia has been described more than 50 years ago [17, 147], few years after the launch of new-generation incubators, leading to more colored (with high FiO_2) premature infants. Immature retinas of premature newborns are sensitive to hyperoxemia, which disrupts neurovascular growth, leading to retinopathy of prematurity [145]. Pathophysiology involves several phases: retinal vasculature is first inhibited due to hyperoxemia and other factors in particular nutritional. The retinal growth will then be done with reduced vascularization, which leads to hypoxemia, which itself stimulates the expression of oxygen-regulated growth factors such as erythropoietin (EPO), VEGF (vascular endothelial growth factor), and IGF1 (insulin-like growth factor), leading to neovascularization [145]. The developing immature brain is particularly sensitive to changes in oxygen and in particular to hyperoxemia, as is well demonstrated in a recent review [146].

1.4   Technical Aspects of Oxygen Delivery

1.4.1   Oxygen Sources

Currently, there are several oxygen sources available: low-pressure oxygen concentrators and liquid oxygen mostly used for home care, pressurized oxygen in cylinders for intrahospital or ambulance transportation, and pressurized medical oxygen mainly used in hospitals. At the beginning of oxygen medical use, the administration of oxygen supposed a local production by the users, as did Beddoes and Watt at the Pneumatic Institution [34, 148]. This explains in part the initially limited medical use of this gas. In 1868, Barth was able to provide almost 60 L (15 gallons) of oxygen compressed with hand pump into a copper bottle [148]. This was enough for intermittent administration of oxygen but larger cylinders of up to 100 gallons were available at the end of the nineteenth century when continuous administration was described [43]. In 1965, the first liquid oxygen system was developed [149] and few years later, the first stationary oxygen concentrators became available [150]. Oxygen concentrators produced a purity of gas of around 90% while hospital oxygen has around 99% purity. The other characteristic of medical air is to be very dry [151, 152] and the question of humidification of this gas is still debated.

1.4.2 Humidification

The question regarding the humidification requirement for low, moderate, and high-flow oxygen is not fully resolved, and recommendations are not homogeneous. The oxygen delivered in hospitals is dry, with less than 5 mgH_2O/L of water content [151, 152] or even less than 1 mgH_2O/L [153]. It is recommended in North America to humidify oxygen when flow rates are above 4 L/min [154, 155] while these recommendations rely on few data. Cold humidification with bubble humidification is expensive and of limited efficacy. The dry oxygen delivered through nasal cannula or non-occlusive mask represents only a fraction of the inspiratory gases in spontaneously breathing patients with respiratory failure, when low or moderate flow is delivered (below 15 L/min). The inspiratory flow during acute respiratory failure is frequently above 60 L/min [156]; this implies that dry medical oxygen is mixed with room air and final FiO_2 as well as humidity at the trachea level is the result from blended FiO_2 and humidity of the medical oxygen and room air. With low to moderate flows, the impact of room air characteristics is probably major, as more than 50% of the inspiratory gas is coming from room air rather than from the medical gas. Consequently, the impact of humidification of the delivered oxygen may be limited (Fig. 1.5). The poor performance of cold humidification to prevent nasal dryness was demonstrated in Chanques et al.'s study for patients managed in ICU with moderate flows (median 7 L/min) as discussed above [151]. It was also shown in 185 patients hospitalized in the ward that there were no or few difference in mucosal dryness symptoms between the use of bubble humidifier and no humidification [157]. The recent British Thoracic Guidelines for oxygen therapy recommend using humidification only for prolonged use of high-flow oxygen therapy but not for low flow delivered with nasal cannulae or mask [13]. In these guidelines, the use of cold humidification (bubble humidifiers) is not recommended considering the lack of demonstration of clinical impact [13].

It was also shown in a randomized controlled trial (RCT) conducted in 18 patients receiving long-term low-flow oxygen therapy that cold bubble humidification did not perform better than no humidification and did not change the impact on outcome or on pulmonary function [158]. In both groups, during a 2-year follow-up, nasal mucociliary clearance and pulmonary function decreased similarly, and local inflammation slightly increased. This study raised the question of active humidification during low-flow long-term oxygen therapy. This issue is discussed in another chapter of this book.

In a recently published randomized controlled trial conducted in 354 ICU patients receiving oxygen with nasal cannula or mask, *no humidification* was compared to

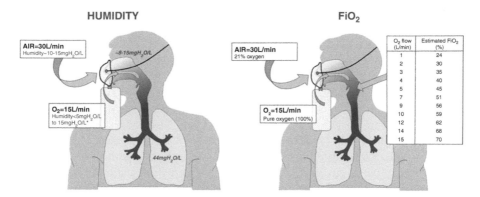

Fig. 1.5 Inspiratory gases during conventional oxygen therapy are a mixture of medical oxygen (dry pure oxygen) and air (21% oxygen with humidity around 10–15 mgH$_2$O/L). The impact of this mixing on humidity (left panel) and FiO$_2$ (right panel) of inspiratory gases is represented. In this example with a mask reservoir providing 15 L/min and a total inspiratory flow of 45 L/min, the FiO$_2$ is about 70%. Maximum FiO$_2$ is always lower than 100% as a part of the inspiratory gas is ambient air. The chart of estimated FiO$_2$ for oxygen flow rate from 1 to 15 L/min is provided [167]. Absolute humidity of air and medical gas is indicated based on published data [151, 152]. Medical gases are dry (below 5 mgH$_2$O/L when nonhumidified and almost 15 mgH$_2$O/L with cold humidification*). The mixture of air and medical gases enters the airways between 8 and 15 mgH$_2$O/L, and is warmed and humidified along the airways to reach 44 mgH$_2$O/L in the alveoli

bubble humidification on comfort, using a 15-item comfort scale [159]. The evaluated hypothesis was the non-inferiority of oxygen therapy without humidification. Most patients received oxygen flow below 4 L/min, and 28% of the patients received higher flows 6–8 h after inclusion. The overall oxygen therapy discomfort was low with or without humidification. After 6–8 h, the study was underpowered to verify the non-inferiority hypothesis. However, differences on comfort were very low between cold humidification and no humidification. The comfort was non-inferior after 24 h for low flow without humidification. In the small subgroup of patients with higher flows, the discomfort was slightly higher after 24 h. Importantly, none of the other important outcomes (need for bronchoscopy, rate of NIV use or intubation, ICU length of stay, and death) differed between groups [159].

Based on these data, the systematic utilization of cold humidification should be avoided for low and moderate oxygen flows (below 15 L/min) when used for less than 24 h. The absence of systematic use of humidification with oxygen therapy is safe and a potential important cost-saving measure.

1.4.3 Interfaces to Deliver Low-Flow Oxygen

Oxygen tents, hoods, oxygen chamber, mouthpiece, facial and nasal masks, pharyngeal catheter, nasal prongs, nasal cannula, nasal cannula with reservoir (mustache) … several type of interfaces have been used to deliver oxygen [148]. Haldane proposed to deliver oxygen via a mask [44], but it was considered a cumbersome method. Nasal cannula's first utilization during the first world war was attributed to captain Adrian Stokes [35] and it has been evaluated by Barach in 1929 [160] and is still the most frequently used interface to deliver oxygen flow rate below 6–8 L/min. If higher flows are required for prolonged time of several hours, other interfaces should be used and humidification may be added [13, 155]. Nasal prongs are also used, especially in neonates. Non-occlusive facial masks are frequently used with higher oxygen flow rates, with or without reservoir. Reservoir should be kept for situations requiring oxygen flows above 10 L/min, and may lead to CO_2 rebreathing if low flow is used [154]. Non-rebreathing masks are used and specific facial mask with open design may lead to reduced oxygen rebreathing, but only few data are available [161]. Venturi masks are also used allowing humidification of the oxygen through nebulization. This device was described by Campbell in 1960 [162].

1.4.4 Estimation of FiO_2 Delivered in Spontaneously Breathing Patients

This question has been extensively discussed and several studies have tried to provide estimation of the delivered FiO_2 in relation with oxygen flow rate. FiO_2 of the inspiratory gas is related to the proportion of pure oxygen coming from the interface (with 100% FiO_2) and from the room air (with 21% FiO_2) (Fig. 1.5). The "real" delivered FiO_2 is then related to several factors such as the interface used to deliver oxygen, the respiratory rate, the minute ventilation, the peak inspiratory flow, and the route of respiration (mouth vs. nose breathers). Studies have found either no difference between mouth-open and mouth-closed breathing [163, 164] or a significantly higher FiO_2 during mouth-closed breathing compared to mouth-open breathing [165, 166] or the opposite [167]. However, these estimations may be helpful to evaluate the patient's needs and severity [168]. It must be kept in mind that even with 15 L/min delivered with an oxygen mask, FiO_2 is usually below 80% and slightly above 70% [167] (Fig. 1.5).

1.4.5 Monitoring of Conventional Oxygen Therapy

Clinical evaluation of patients receiving oxygen therapy is essential, including respiratory rate, signs of respiratory distress, and other vital parameters. In addition, a monitoring of several other parameters is now recommended for patients receiving conventional oxygen therapy, and pulse oximetry (SpO_2) should be used "in all breathless and acutely ill patients" [13]. British Thoracic Society also recommends to monitor a physiological "track and trigger" system such as the national early warning score (NEWS) [13, 169].

Pulse oximetry is usually sufficient for oxygenation monitoring and even if differences exist between devices, it is usually considered that several oximeters from different leading companies are equivalent in terms of accuracy for SpO_2 values above 80%, when tested in optimal conditions with healthy subjects [170–172].

However, when the comparisons are conducted in patients, differences between oximeters are more pronounced [173–176]. In patients with suspected increased $PaCO_2$ (in patients with suspected or known CO_2 retention and especially in the case of loss of consciousness) and in patients with suspected metabolic disorders (renal insufficiency, shock states, or in specific intoxications), arterial blood gas analysis with lactate dosage may be required initially then based on patient clinical evolution [13]. Arterial blood gases are mainly used to measure pH, $PaCO_2$, and bicarbonates. Indeed, especially if oxygenation recommendations are followed (i.e., if SpO_2 is maintained between 88 and 92% or 90 and 94%), the PaO_2 values are not required. The prescription of long-term oxygen therapy may be an exception and PaO_2 may be required to decide on the initiation of this treatment [177]. In other situations, capillary blood gases may be sufficient for clinician decisions and preferred for patient's comfort [178]. A meta-analysis of the study comparing these measurement techniques, pH, $PaCO_2$, and bicarbonate values was well correlated with arterial and capillary blood gases [179].

Concerning oximetry measurements there are well-known limitations (dyshemo-globinemia, polish nail, pigmented skin, low perfusion, motion artifact …) [180, 181]. Inaccuracies of oximeters are frequently reported in the case of low SpO_2 (below 80%) and in the case of pigmented skins [170, 171]. However, technical improvement has improved accuracy in difficult situations. It was shown by Jubran and Tobin in 1990 that in populations with pigmented skin, SpO_2 above 95% was required to obtain sufficient oxygenation [182]. Currently, with recent oximeters, these differences among the devices are small within usual levels of SpO_2. During severe hypoxemia, however, a gap between SaO_2 and SpO_2 of several percentage may exists. In Binkler and Feiner studies, with pigmented skins, oximeters overestimated SpO_2 by 2.5–5% in comparison with SaO_2, especially at very low values (below 70%) and with large standard deviations [170, 171, 173]. Within well-recognized companies for pulse oximetry (Masimo, Nonin, and Nellcor) Fiener et al. showed that the bias with reference values (SaO_2) was low whatever the color of the skin when SaO_2/SpO_2 values were above 80% [171]. In this study, bias of plus or minus 4% still existed with very low SpO_2 values (60–70%) and differences up to 10% could be detected in SpO_2 values among the tested devices during severe hypoxemia, especially when disposable sensor was used [171]. Yamamoto et al. showed that polish nail had only minor impact of SpO_2 measurements [183]. In a study conducted in 33 healthy females, several colors were tested and authors found moderately reduced SpO_2 values with specific colors (blue, beige, purple, and white) but tested oximeters were not among the reference oximeters [184].

Scoring systems have been developed for the early recognition of patients at risk for clinical deterioration [185]. Many scores have been developed (EWS, MEWS, NEWS, ViEWS, AbEWS, NEWS2, NEWS-L [186–189] …). Currently there are more than 100 different published track and trigger systems [190], most of which have been modified from the original Early Warning Score [189] developed using expert opinion, and have demonstrated variable levels of reliability, validity, and usefulness [191]. Meta-analyses have been conducted to evaluate the impact of the implementation of these scores on outcome [185]. The national early warning score (NEWS), which uses physiological parameters for scoring, may be beneficial for predicting patient deterioration [189]. However, a general conclusion cannot be generated due to the heterogeneity of the score used in the studies and the use in different populations [192]. The monitoring of early warning scores (Early Warning Score (EWS), National Early Warning Score (NEWS), or other scores) has been recommended [13, 169]. When compared to quick sepsis-related organ failure assessment (qSOFA) and systemic inflammatory response syndrome (SIRS), NEWS was found to be the most accurate for the detection of all sepsis endpoints [193, 194]. The introduction of the NEWS did not change the patient outcome in several recent evaluations [195, 196]. NEWS can predict outcome and discriminate patients' severity when evaluated at the emergency department and after admission [197].

Clinical events before in-hospital cardiac arrest are mainly respiratory events with increased respiratory rate [198]. Respiratory rate is among the first vital signs to change in deteriorating patients and it has been reported to be the best individual predictor of cardiac arrest in general wards [199]. However, the usual vital parameters, including SpO_2 values and respiratory rate, are insufficiently monitored in the general ward in patients before severe outcomes (cardiac arrest, ICU admission, or unexpected death) [200, 201].

In comparison with the preexisting EWS models, the S/F ratio showed better or comparable predictive accuracy for unexpected ICU transfers in the respiratory wards [202]. With automated oxygen titration devices, the parameters of oxygenation and respiratory parameters are continuously monitored and "respiratory scores" such as $EWS.O_2$ including these parameters and trends may be helpful to monitor the patients receiving oxygen therapy but additional results are required (Fig. 1.6) [203, 204].

1.5   Devices Available to Deliver Oxygen in Spontaneously Breathing Patients

We will discuss below the devices to deliver low or moderate oxygen flows (<15 L/min). High-flow nasal therapy systems are described in other chapters.

In hospitals, oxygen supplementation is provided from a high-pressure source and a pressure regulator first reduces the working pressure of the gas to around 50 psi [205]. The most common device to titrate oxygen is the rotameter or oxygen flowmeter that has been used for more than one century, as the first publication for medical use was in 1910 [21, 206]. Clinicians do the titration manually. Oxygen flowmeters usually deliver flow from 0 to 5 or 0 to 10 L/min, but some devices may provide higher flows; at flush setting, these devices deliver up to 60 L/min [205]. The other conventional way to titrate oxygen is through Venturi mask [162], with which clinicians manually set an estimated FiO_2 from 21 to 100%. However, it is usually considered that real FiO_2 may not be higher than 70% especially in patients with high respiratory drives leading to high inspiratory flows higher than 60 L/min during hypoxemic respiratory failure [156].

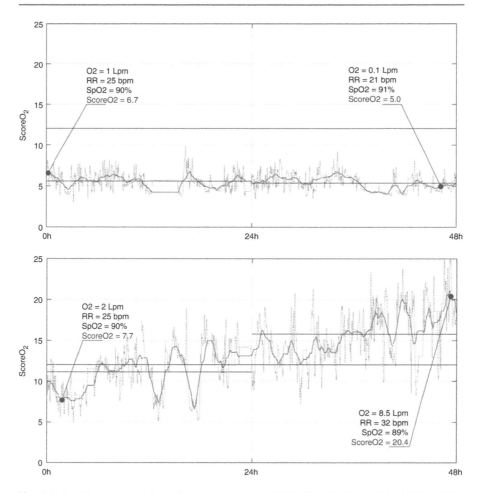

Fig. 1.6 Continuous evaluation of a respiratory score (Early Warning Score.O_2) with FreeO$_2$ in spontaneously breathing patients to monitor respiratory severity. The continuous measurement of SpO$_2$, oxygen flow rate, respiratory rate, and heart rate as well as other derived parameters allows continuous display of severity scores based on important clinical parameters. The respiratory score during 48 h of a patient with good clinical evolution is shown on the upper panel. This patient was discharged from the hospital the next day. The respiratory score during 48 h of a patient with deterioration of the clinical condition leading to ICU transfer and endotracheal intubation is shown on the lower panel. Oxygen flow rate (O$_2$), pulse oximetry (SpO$_2$), and respiratory rate (RR) at the beginning and end of the recordings are provided. SpO$_2$ target was set at 90% on FreeO$_2$

1.5.1 Innovations in Oxygen Delivery

1.5.1.1 Automated Adjustment of Oxygen Therapy

The difficulty of the knowledge transfer is partly related to resistance to changing habits and limited knowledge [207]. These two aspects may explain the failure to implement oxygen recommendations [8, 208]. Austin et al. compared usual oxygen with a new protocol to manually titrate O_2 flow rate to maintain SpO_2 target at 88–92% [5]. Noncompliance with the oxygen titration protocol involved 56% of the patients, even if patients were part of a randomized controlled trial. This reflects the difficulties to change the practices, even if the complications related to hyperoxemia in COPD patients have been known for 70 years [16]. This problem with compliance to oxygen guidelines was shown in different settings [3, 19, 20]. In addition, the implementation of new protocols requires a lot of energy and motivation, as well as frequent and renewed training. Trainings, educational sessions, oxygen alert stickers with protocol reminders, implementation of local guidelines, emails, and other type of interventions have shown to slightly improve the adherence to oxygen protocols [19]. Improvement of adherence to oxygen protocols is achieved after education interventions but declines to pre-intervention levels over time [54]. Despite more than 50 years of trying to transfer knowledge concerning oxygen therapy recommendations, it is possible to conclude that it has failed. New and frequent guidelines [13, 14] may improve the practices; however, first recommendations were published 60 years ago [46] with poor intake from clinicians.

It is well documented that prescription practices for oxygen supplementation and adherence to prescriptions are very poor, probably reflecting unawareness about the necessity of accurate oxygen prescription and therapy [19]. An audit conducted in 2013 by the British Thoracic Society found that only 55% of patients who were administered oxygen during an admission had a written prescription [209]. Despite the low rate of prescription, this was an improvement compared to 2008, where only 32% of patients supplied with oxygen had a written prescription. In an Australian audit, only 3% of inpatients with an exacerbation of COPD had a written oxygen prescription while 79% of the patients received oxygen supplementation [210]. In a large European audit in 2010–2011 of 16,018 patients with an exacerbation in COPD, it was found that 10.1% received inappropriate oxygen therapy, either with high-flow oxygen or no oxygen despite being hypoxemic [211].

One solution is to automate the transfer of knowledge when feasible. In the situation of oxygen therapy, relatively simple and repetitive tasks are involved: measurement of oxygenation and action based on this measurement. Oxygen therapy is quite simple: to increase oxygen when oxygenation is too low and decrease oxygen when it is too high. Closed loops have been previously used for much more complex procedures such as automated weaning from mechanical ventilation [212, 213] or fully automated mechanical ventilation [214, 215]. The closed-loop oxygen adjustment is very suitable and several systems have been developed recently to try to achieve this goal [22–25].

1.5.1.2 Clinical Evaluations Conducted with FreeO₂ (Automated Oxygen Titration)

A new device (FreeO₂™, Quebec, Canada) has been developed which regulates in a closed loop and every second the oxygen flow rate (from 0 to 20 L/min with steps of 0.1 L/min) is administered in spontaneous breathing patients via nasal cannulae or mask, according to a SpO_2 target chosen by the clinician (Fig. 1.7). This system allows, in addition to the precise regulation of oxygen flow rates, to

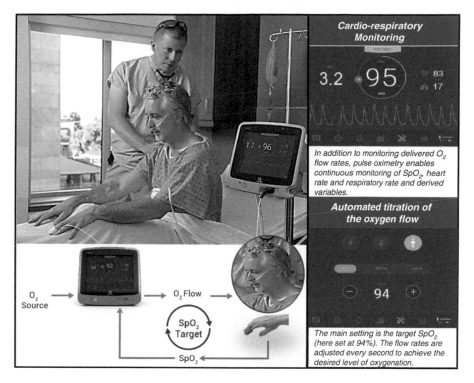

Fig. 1.7 Automated titration devices share the same working principles: an adjustment of the oxygen flow rate to maintain the set SpO_2 target. SpO_2 is continuously measured and oxygen flow is continuously modified according to the difference between the measured and the targeted SpO_2. Continuous monitoring of various parameters is allowed with these devices

monitor important cardiorespiratory parameters: SpO_2, O_2 flow rate, respiratory rate, and heart rate [24]. Initial assessment was carried out mainly in Quebec and France in more than 1000 patients. The $FreeO_2$ algorithm was validated and refined in a study in healthy volunteers with moderate induced hypoxemia conditions [24] and during NIV [216], in COPD patients during walking [217, 218] and during acute exacerbations [219–221], in patients with lung fibrosis during walking [222], in patients with acute myocardial infarction [223], at the emergency department in hypoxemic patients and hypercapnic patients [220], in pediatric patients [224], during central apnea [225], and in patients after thoracic or abdominal surgery [226, 227] (Tables 1.1 and 1.2).

An evaluation of $FreeO_2$ was conducted in 50 hospitalized patients for acute exacerbation of COPD [219]. The study showed the feasibility of using the $FreeO_2$ system for prolonged periods (up to 15 days continuously). The time patients were within the SpO_2 target prescribed by the pulmonologist was $81 \pm 16\%$ with $FreeO_2$ and $51 \pm 20\%$ with manual adjustment, with a significantly shorter duration of desaturation defined by SpO_2 below 85% (0.2% vs. 2.3%, $p < 0.001$) and hyperoxemia, defined by SpO_2 of at least +5% above the target (1.4% vs. 10.4%, $p < 0.001$)

Table 1.1 Clinical evaluations of the automated oxygen titration devices adapted for spontaneously breathing patients. Studies conducted with FreeO$_2$

Studies, References	n	Population	Study design	Main results
			STUDIES CONDUCTED WITH FreeO$_2$	
FreeO$_2$ in healthy subjects (dynamic induced hypoxemia) (ref.24)	10	Healthy subjects	*Cross over RCT* FreeO$_2$ vs. Air vs. continuous O$_2$	With FreeO$_2$, more time in the SpO$_2$ target Less desaturation, less hyperoxia, less induced tachycardia
FreeO$_2$ during NIV and CPAP in healthy subjects (dynamic induced hypoxemia) (ref.216)	10	Healthy subjects	*Cross over RCT* FreeO$_2$ vs. Air vs. continuous O$_2$	With FreeO$_2$, more time in the SpO$_2$ target, less desaturation, less hyperoxia No workload with FreeO$_2$
FreeO$_2$ in COPD patients during endurance shuttle walking (ref.217)	16	COPD patients with desaturation during effort	*Cross over RCT* FreeO$_2$ vs. Air vs. continuous O$_2$	With FreeO$_2$, more time in the SpO$_2$ target, less desaturation, less hyperoxia Increased exercise tolerance vs air (P<0.05). Non significant increase of exercise tolerance vs O$_2$ (P=0.22)
FreeO$_2$ in hypercapnic COPD patients during endurance shuttle walking (ref.218)	12	Severe hypercapnic COPD patients with LTOT	*Cross over RCT* FreeO$_2$ vs. continuous O$_2$	With FreeO$_2$, more time in the SpO$_2$ target, less desaturation, less hyperoxia Increased exercise tolerance vs O$_2$ (P=0.02). No induced hypercapnia
FreeO$_2$ in COPD patients hospitalized for exacerbation (pilot) (ref.219)	50	COPD patients with acute exacerbation	*RCT* FreeO$_2$ vs. continuous O$_2$ (manual setting)	FreeO$_2$ well accepted by care givers and patients (80%) Better oxygenation with FreeO$_2$: more time in the SpO$_2$ target 81 vs. 51%, less time with hyperoxia: 1.5 vs. 10.4% , less time with hypoxemia: 0.2 vs. 2.3% 30% reduction in hospital LOS (5.8 vs. 8.4 days, P=0.051)
Economic evaluation of FreeO$_2$ during acute exacerbation of COPD (ref.228)	47	COPD patients with acute exacerbation	*Economic evaluation* Cost analysis and incremental cost-effectiveness ratios (ICERs)	*Cost analysis* = with FreeO$_2$, -20.7% per-patient costs reduction at 180 days (-Can$ 2,959.71; P=0.13) *ICERs* = FreeO$_2$ savings of -Can$ 96.91 per % point of time spent at the target SpO$_2$
FreeO$_2$ in the ED in patients with ARF (ref.220)	190	ARF in the ED (Hypoxemic and hypercapnic)	*RCT* FreeO$_2$ vs. continuous O$_2$ (manual setting) (Study duration = 3 hours)	Better oxygenation with FreeO$_2$: more time in the SpO$_2$ target 81 vs. 52%, less time with hyperoxia: 4.2 vs. 21.6% , less time with hypoxemia: 3.2 vs. 5.1% More O$_2$ modifications (6715 vs. 3) , more patients weaned for O$_2$ Reduced complications (ICU), reduced hospital LOS (9.2 vs. 11.1 days, P<0.001)
FreeO$_2$ during acute coronary syndrom (pilot) (ref.223)	60	Acute coronary syndrome	*RCT* FreeO$_2$ (target 92%) FreeO$_2$ (target 96%) vs. continuous O$_2$ (manual setting)	Better oxygenation with FreeO$_2$ (time in the target, hyperoxia, hypoxemia) Less time with severe hypoxemia (SpO$_2$ <85%) Less ventricular arythmias
FreeO$_2$ in pediatric patients (bronchiolitis and ARF) (pilot) (ref.224)	60	2 pediatric populations: -Bronchiolitis (1-2 yrs old) -Hypoxemic respiratory distress (2-15 yrs old)	*RCT* FreeO$_2$ vs. continuous O$_2$ (manual setting) (Study duration = 6 hours)	95% of the time in the SpO$_2$ target with FreeO$_2$ vs.76% with manual setting Better oxygenation (time in the target, hyperoxia, hypoxemia) Reduced hospital LOS
FreeO$_2$ in patients with idiopathic lung fibrosis during exercise (ref.222)	16	Severe IPF	*Two consecutive 6MWT* continuous O$_2$ - FreeO$_2$	Less desaturation end of 6MWT (87.4% vs 83.5%, P=0.039), Less dyspnea (Borg=6.3 vs 4.8, P=0.02). Increased exercise tolerance vs O$_2$ (309 vs. 252 m, P=0.016)
FreeO$_2$ during induced cyclic desaturations (model of central apnea) (ref.61)	5	Healthy subjects	*RCT* FreeO$_2$ (2 different controls) vs. continuous O$_2$ (2 and 4 L/min) vs. Air during cyclic desaturations	With FreeO$_2$, more time in the SpO$_2$ target (92%) Less desaturation in comparison with air, Less hyperoxia in comparison with constant O$_2$ Reduced O$_2$ consumption in comparison with continuous O$_2$
FreeO$_2$ last generation (ref.225)	50	COPD patients with acute exacerbation	*Two consecutive recorded periods* Continuous O$_2$ (30 minutes) followed by FreeO$_2$ (60 minutes) followed by FreeO$_2$ up to 3 days	With FreeO$_2$, reduction of O$_2$ flow rate from 2 to 1L/min (P=0.01), increased time in the SpO$_2$ target (53 vs. 84% of the time, P<0.05), hyperoxemia and severe hypoxemia <1% of the time improved comfort with wireless oximeter (P=0.003)
FreeO$_2$ post-op patients (ref.227)	198	Adult patients with abdominal or thoracic surgery at risk of complications.	*RCT* FreeO$_2$ vs. continuous O$_2$ (manual setting) Analyses during 3 hours (revovery room) and during 3 days after surgery	With FreeO$_2$, more time in the SpO$_2$ target (91 vs. 40%) after 3 hours (recovery room) and after 3 days post-surgery (94 vs. 62%) Less desaturation (2 vs. 5 min) and hyperoxia (12 vs. 97 min) in comparison with manual O$_2$ (recovery room) Less desaturation (31 vs. 373 min) and hyperoxia (148 vs. 800 min) in comparison with manual O$_2$ (3 days post surgery) Less patients with oxygen after 3 days with FreeO$_2$ (18 vs. 33%)
FreeO$_2$ in ICU patients (ref.229)	51	Adult patients in the ICU after mechanical ventilation weaning	*Prospective crossover cohort study* O$_2$ parameters and O$_2$ consumption were recorded during constant O$_2$ flow (30 minutes) and FreeO$_2$ modes (2 hours)	SpO$_2$ range was significantly higher with FreeO$_2$ mode compared to constant O$_2$ flow mode [87% vs. 43%; p < 0.001]. Time with hyperoxia was lower with FreeO$_2$ mode: 8.7% vs. 38.3% Total O$_2$ consumption was lower with FreeO$_2$: 120 vs. 240 L/min, P<0.001
FreeO$_2$ in COVID-19 patients (submitted)	59	Adult patients with COVID-19	*Prospective observationnal study* 21 patients after weaning from MV, 7 after high-flow nasal therapy, 31 as a first-line therapy.	Time within SpO$_2$ target = 86.3±10.6% Time within hypoxemia = 1.3±2.8% Time with hyperoxaemia = 2.8±6.2%

Table 1.2 Clinical evaluations of the automated oxygen titration devices adapted for spontaneously breathing patients. Studies conducted with other closed-loop systems

Studies, References	n	Population	assessed.	Main results
			STUDIES CONDUCTED WITH other oxygen closed-loops	
O$_2$ flow regulator during exercise in COPD patients with LTOT (ref.22)	18	COPD patients with LTOT	*Cross over RCT* O$_2$ flow regulator vs. continuous O$_2$ 15 minutes constant load cycling exercise	There were no differences in symptoms or heart rate With O$_2$ flow regulator: higher SpO$_2$ (95 vs. 93%, P=0.04) Less time below the target SpO$_2$ (171 vs. 340 seconds, P<0.001) Less therapist time (5.6 vs. 2.0 minutes, P<0.005)
AccuO$_2$™, Closed-Loop Oxygen Conserving Device for Stable COPD Patients (ref.25)	22	COPD patients with LTOT	*Cross over RCT* AccuO$_2$™ vs. continuous O$_2$ vs. continuous O$_2$ device during 8 hours/day, 2 days	Mean SpO$_2$ was 90.7 with AccuO$_2$™ vs. 92.2 %, P<0.005 Compared to continuous O$_2$ with AccuO$_2$™, conservation ratios were 9.9 with AccuO$_2$™ and 2.6 for conserving O$_2$ device, P< 0.001 with AccuO$_2$™, non significant reduction of hypoxemia Significant increased time with SpO$_2$ >90%
O$_2$matic® during admission with exacerbation of COPD (ref.26)	19	COPD patients with acute exacerbation	*Cross over RCT* O$_2$matic® vs. continuous O$_2$ 4 hours with each strategy	With O$_2$matic®, better oxygenation: increased time in the target 85 vs. 47%, P=0.01 reduced time with severe hypoxia 1.3 vs. 18%, P=0.01 reduced time with hyperoxia 4.6 vs. 10.5%, P=0.2
O$_2$matic® in COVID-19 patients (ref.232)	15	COVID-19 patients in the medical ward	*Prospective observationnal study*	SpO$_2$ in the target 82.9% of the time. Time with hypoxemia (SpO$_2$ > 2% below target) = 5.1% Time with hyperexemia (SpO$_2$ > 2% above target) = 0.6%.

with automated adjustment in comparison with manual adjustment. The duration of hospitalization was 5.8 ± 4.4 days with FreeO$_2$ vs. 8.4 ± 6.0 days with manual adjustment ($p = 0.051$) [219]. A cost-effectiveness study has demonstrated, taking into account the cost of the technology, with a reduction in costs of 21.6% (−3091$

in Canadian dollars) at 180 days. The study demonstrated that this technology is cost effective for all oxygenation criteria [228].

A multicenter randomized study compared manual titration or FreeO$_2$ at the emergency department [220]. One hundred ninety patients admitted to the emergency department for acute respiratory distress requiring oxygen were included and randomized to receive oxygen for 3 h with manual or automated titration [220]. In the FreeO$_2$ group, there were fewer desaturations, less hyperoxemia, and more time in the SpO$_2$ target. In addition, more patients were completely (14.1% vs. 4.3%, $p < 0.001$) or partially (more than 50% decrease O$_2$, 30% vs. 17%, $p < 0.001$) weaned from O$_2$ during the 3-h study period. Despite a limited duration of exposure to 3 h, there was an impact beyond the study period: the duration of oxygen administration in the hospital was reduced (5.6 vs. 7.1 days, $p = 0.002$) and the length of stay was significantly reduced (9.2 vs. 11.1 days, $p = 0.001$) in the FreeO$_2$ group.

Oxygen strategy has been evaluated in 198 postoperative patients, with 103 randomized to usual oxygen titration and 95 randomized to automated oxygen titration [227]. Time in the SpO$_2$ range was higher in the automated group, both initially ($\leqslant$3 h; 91.4% vs. 40.2% of time, $p < 0.0001$) and during the 3-day period (94.0% vs. 62.1% of time, $p < 0.0001$). Periods of hypoxemia were reduced in the automated group (33 min vs. 370 min), as well as hyperoxemia under oxygen (5 min vs. 178 min, $p < 0.0001$). Oxygen was still prescribed after day 3 in 33.3% versus 18.3% of patients in the standard and automated groups, respectively ($p = 0.01$) [227].

Recently, FreeO$_2$ was evaluated in Tunisia in 51 ICU patients after extubation during 2 h [229]. The time in the SpO$_2$ target increased twofold with automated oxygen titration (87% vs. 43% of the time, $p < 0.001$), while oxygen consumption decreased twofold in comparison with usual titration (121 vs. 240 L/h, $p < 0.001$) [229]. Reduction of oxygen use has also been evaluated with automated oxygen titration in 36 hospitalized patients on oxygen therapy. SpO$_2$ targets at 90, 92, 94, 96, and 98% were set and oxygen flow at steady state was collected [230]. The mean oxygen flow increased twofold from 90% to 92% of SpO$_2$ target and increased by a factor of 6.3 from 90% to 98%.

A meta-analysis described the benefits on oxygenation, hospital length of stay, and duration of oxygen therapy but authors concluded that other data are necessary [231].

1.5.1.3 Other Systems Allowing Automatic Adjustment of Oxygen

Three studies have been published to evaluate other devices using a closed loop between SpO$_2$ and oxygen flow rates [22, 25, 26]. In one study, the authors evaluated a closed-loop oxygen-adjusting system (O$_2$ Flow Regulator, Dima, Bologna, Italy) during exercise in 18 oxygen-dependent COPD patients [22]. The device was set to maintain SpO$_2$ at 94%. Mean SpO$_2$ was 95 ± 2% with automated adjustment and 93 ± 3% with manual adjustment ($p = 0.04$). Patients spent significantly less time below the target SpO$_2$ (171 ± 187 s vs. 340 ± 220 s, $p < 0.001$) with the O$_2$ Flow Regulator. The manual intervention time decreased with the automated adjustment (2.0 ± 0.1 vs. 5.6 ± 3.7 min, $p = 0.005$). In another published study, Rice et al. evaluated a closed-loop device to titrate oxygen (AccuO$_2$™, OptiSat Medical, Inc.

Minneapolis, USA) in 28 COPD patients with long-term oxygen therapy [25]. The closed loop was compared to constant oxygen flow and to an O_2-conserving device. The mean SpO_2 was significantly different at 90.7 ± 1.9% (AccuO$_2$™) vs. 92.4 ± 3.6% vs. 92.2 ± 4.4% compared to traditional oxygen delivery systems [25]. In addition, this system reduced oxygen consumption with oxygen retention ratios of 9.9 ± 7.3 and 2.6 ± 1.0 compared to other oxygen delivery systems ($p < 0.001$) [25]. Recently, Hansen et al. evaluated a new closed loop (O2matic, O2matic Ltd., Herlev, Denmark) in 19 COPD patients hospitalized for exacerbation. Patients were managed in crossover randomly with manual or automated oxygen titration during 4 h. During automated titration, SpO_2 was maintained in the target 85.1% of the time vs. 46.6% with manually controlled oxygen ($p < 0.001$). Time with $SpO_2 < 85\%$ was 1.3% with automated titration and 17.9% with manual oxygen titration ($p = 0.01$). Time with SpO_2 above target did not differ (4.6% vs. 10.5%, $p = 0.2$) [26]. Recently, O2matic has been evaluated in an observational study on 15 patients with COVID-19 [232]. The device was used during a mean of 2.7 days and patients were in the SpO_2 target at a mean of 82.9% of time, 12.0% of the time below the target, and 5.1% of the time above the target [232]. Several aspects such as range flows, accuracy, and type of control differ when comparing the available devices [22, 25, 26]. No comparison has been conducted so far comparing the existing systems. Other devices have been developed for intubated premature infants and will not be discussed here [23].

The potential benefits of the automated system to titrate oxygen exist for both patients (better control of oxygenation, better monitoring) than for the health system (reduction of workload, better follow-up of recommendations, strategies integrating telemedicine, cost savings) [233, 234].

These systems could improve the management of COPD patients across the continuum of care [235] and for other populations than accurate oxygen titration [14]. During the initial management of COPD exacerbations, automated oxygen adjustment based on recommendations should improve the outcome of these patients by reducing the frequency and severity of respiratory acidosis [106, 108]. By combining telemedicine with automated oxygen titration, new management strategies for COPD patients can be envisaged, which should make it possible to shorten the length of hospital stays and thus the overall cost of treating these patients.

1.6   Conclusion

Conventional oxygen therapy is used daily by most of the clinicians in hospitals and is one of the most common drug, but knowledge about its toxicity remains limited and overlooked. The main belief is that oxygen is a vital gas and that it can not be harmful while literature is compelling and now demonstrates that hyperoxemia increases morbidity and mortality in populations daily managed with liberal oxygen in hospitals and beyond. Both aspects of this gas (vital and toxic) should now be considered and recent recommendations underline that hypoxemia as well as hyperoxemia are detrimental to patients. Severe hypoxemia may be an immediate threat for the patients while hyperoxemia, while less visible, may be as dangerous with systemic, vascular, and cellular impacts. In premature infants and in COPD the need to accurately titrate oxygen has been known for a long time but it is difficult to achieve. In other populations, accurate titration of oxygen during hospitalization is also mandatory. The first goal of oxygen therapy is to treat hypoxemia, and the other major goal is to avoid hyperoxemia. In COPD patients, oxygen flow rate should be titrated to maintain SpO_2 between 88 and 92%. In other populations, it is now recommended to maintain SpO_2 values in a tight range between 90 and 94%. Situations with SpO_2 values above the target such as values below the target should be considered as dangerous for the patients. There is no room anymore for hyperox(em)ia in the healthcare system [9, 236]! The knowledge transfer concerning oxygen therapy seems to be a failure. Similarly to other areas in medicine, automated knowledge transfer by using closed-loop systems could be a solution. Current systems to manually adjust oxygen flow, "oxygen flowmeters" use the principle of rotameter, a more than centenary technology [21, 206]. For a century, few innovations have been occurring in the field of oxygen therapy, yet technological improvements allow the use of more sophisticated devices to accurately titrate the oxygen flow rate, to improve efficiency, safety, and monitoring. These automated systems may be useful in many clinical settings such as COPD but also beyond, and initial assessments of these devices demonstrate their potential impact.

Acknowledgements Competing interests: François Lellouche and Erwan L'Her are co-founders, shareholders, and directors of OxyNov. This research and development company has designed and marketed the automated oxygen adjustment system (FreeO$_2$) mentioned in the manuscript.

References

1. Papazian L, et al. Use of high-flow nasal cannula oxygenation in ICU adults: a narrative review. Intensive Care Med. 2016;42(9):1336–49.
2. O'Driscoll BR, et al. British Thoracic Society emergency oxygen audits. Thorax. 2011;66(8): 734–5.
3. Hale KE, Gavin C, O'Driscoll BR. Audit of oxygen use in emergency ambulances and in a hospital emergency department. Emerg Med J. 2008;25(11):773–6.
4. *The National Confidential Enquiry into Patient Outcome and Death. Inspiring Change. 2017. London* 2017.
5. Austin MA, et al. Effect of high flow oxygen on mortality in chronic obstructive pulmonary disease patients in prehospital setting: randomised controlled trial. BMJ. 2010;341: c5462.
6. Chu DK, et al. Mortality and morbidity in acutely ill adults treated with liberal versus conservative oxygen therapy (IOTA): a systematic review and meta-analysis. Lancet. 2018;391(10131):1693–705.
7. Girardis M, et al. Effect of conservative vs conventional oxygen therapy on mortality among patients in an intensive care unit: the oxygen-ICU randomized clinical trial. JAMA. 2016;316(15):1583–9.
8. Beasley R, et al. High-concentration oxygen therapy in COPD. Lancet. 2011;378(9795):969–70.
9. McEvoy JW. Excess oxygen in acute illness: adding fuel to the fire. Lancet. 2018;391(10131): 1640–2.

10. Lellouche F. Oxygen for myocardial infarction: not an open Bar! JACC Cardiovasc Interv. 2018;11(16):1598–600.
11. O'Driscoll BR, et al. A study of attitudes, beliefs and organisational barriers related to safe emergency oxygen therapy for patients with COPD (chronic obstructive pulmonary disease) in clinical practice and research. BMJ Open Respir Res. 2016;3(1):e000102.
12. Burls A, et al. Oxygen use in acute myocardial infarction: an online survey of health professionals' practice and beliefs. Emerg Med J. 2010;27:283–6.
13. O'Driscoll BR, et al. BTS guideline for oxygen use in adults in healthcare and emergency settings. Thorax. 2017;72(Suppl 1):ii1–ii90.
14. Siemieniuk RAC, et al. Oxygen therapy for acutely ill medical patients: a clinical practice guideline. BMJ. 2018;363:k4169.
15. Sjoberg F, Singer M. The medical use of oxygen: a time for critical reappraisal. J Intern Med. 2013;274(6):505–28.
16. Davies CE, Mackinnon J. Neurological effects of oxygen in chronic cor pulmonale. Lancet. 1949;2(6585):883–5. illust
17. Terry TL. Extreme prematurity and fibroblastic overgrowth of persistent vascular sheath behind each crystalline lens. Am J Ophthalmol. 1942;25:203–4.
18. Patz A, Hoeck LE, De La Cruz E. Studies on the effect of high oxygen administration in retrolental fibroplasia. I. Nursery observations. Am J Ophthalmol. 1952;35(9): 1248–53.
19. Cousins JL, Wark PA, McDonald VM. Acute oxygen therapy: a review of prescribing and delivery practices. Int J Chron Obstruct Pulmon Dis. 2016;11:1067–75.
20. Ringbaek TJ, Terkelsen J, Lange P. Outcomes of acute exacerbations in COPD in relation to pre-hospital oxygen therapy. Eur Clin Respir J. 2015;2
21. Foregger R. The rotameter and the waterwheel. Anaesthesist. 2001;50:701–8.
22. Cirio S, Nava S. Pilot study of a new device to titrate oxygen flow in hypoxic patients on long-term oxygen therapy. Respir Care. 2011;56(4):429–34.
23. Claure N, Bancalari E. Automated closed loop control of inspired oxygen concentration. Respir Care. 2013;58(1):151–61.
24. Lellouche F, L'Her E. Automated oxygen flow titration to maintain constant oxygenation. Respir Care. 2012;57(8):1254–62.
25. Rice KL, et al. A portable, closed-loop oxygen conserving device for stable COPD patients: comparison with fixed dose delivery systems. Respir Care. 2011;
26. Hansen EF, et al. Automated oxygen control with O2matic® during admission with exacerbation of COPD. Int J COPD. 2018;13:3997–4003.
27. Heffner JE. The story of oxygen. Respir Care. 2013;58(1):18–31.
28. Prinke RT. New light on the alchemical writings of Michael Sendivogius (1566–1636). Ambix. 2016;63(3):217–43.
29. Lavoisier A-L. Mémoire sur la combustion en général. Mémoires de l'Académie des Sciences, 1777: p. 593.
30. Holmes Frédéric L. The boundaries of Lavoisier's chemical revolution /Les limites de la révolution chimique de Lavoisier. Débats et chantiers actuels autour de Lavoisier et de la révolution chimique. Revue d'histoire des Sciences. 1995;48(1–2):9–48.
31. Priestley J. Experiments and observations on different kinds of air, vol. 101. 2nd ed. London: J. Johnson; 1775.
32. Caillens, Observations sur un nouveau moyen de remedier à la phtisie pulmonaire. Gazette de Santé, 1783: p. 38.
33. Beddoes T, Watt J. Considerations on the medicinal use, and on the production of factitious airs. Ann Med. 1796:245–65.
34. Leigh JM. Early treatment with oxygen. The pneumatic institute and the panaceal literature of the nineteenth century. Anaesthesia. 1974;29(2):194–208.
35. Grainge C. Breath of life: the evolution of oxygen therapy. J R Soc Med. 2004;97(10):489–93.
36. Smith AH. Oxygen gas as a remedy in disease. New York: D. Appleton & Company; 1870.
37. Haldane JS. Respiration. London: Oxford University Press; 1922.

38. Barcroft JR. Supply of oxygen to the tissues. The scientific monthly, vol. 11. New York: The Science Press; 1920.
39. Christiansen J, Douglas CG, Haldane JS. The absorption and dissociation of carbon dioxide by human blood. J Physiol. 1914;48(4):244–71.
40. Jobling MA. The unexpected always happens. Investig Genet. 2012;3:5.
41. Clark R. The life and work of JBS Haldane Oxford: Oxford University Press; 1968.
42. Barach AL. The therapeutic use of oxygen. JAMA. 1922;79(9):693–8.
43. Blodgett AN. The continuous inhalation of oxygen in cases of pneumonia otherwise fatal, and in other diseases. Boston Med Surg J. 1890;123:481–4.
44. Haldane JS. The therapeutic administration of oxygen. Br Med J. 1917;1(2928):181–3.
45. Haldane JS. A lecture on the symptoms, causes, and prevention of Anoxaemia (insufficient supply of oxygen to the tissues), and the value of oxygen in its treatment. Br Med J. 1919;2(3055):65–71.
46. Campbell EJ. Respiratory failure: the relation between oxygen concentrations of inspired air and arterial blood. Lancet. 1960;2(7140):10–1.
47. Massaro DJ, Katz S, Luchsinger PC. Effect of various modes of oxygen administration on the arterial gas values in patients with respiratory acidosis. Br Med J. 1962;2(5305):627–9.
48. Leigh JM. Oxygen therapy techniques after 200 years. A survey of present practice and current trends. Anaesthesia. 1973;28(2):164–9.
49. Jouneau S, et al. Management of acute exacerbations of chronic obstructive pulmonary disease (COPD). Guidelines from the Societe de pneumologie de langue francaise (summary). Rev Mal Respir. 2017;34(4):282–322.
50. Beasley R, et al. Thoracic Society of Australia and new Zealand oxygen guidelines for acute oxygen use in adults: 'Swimming between the flags'. Respirology. 2015;20(8):1182–91.
51. Group, B.I.U.K.C, et al. Oxygen saturation and outcomes in preterm infants. N Engl J Med. 2013;368(22):2094–104.
52. Thein OS, et al. Oxygen prescription: improving compliance using methods from BMJ open quality journal. BMJ Open Qual. 2018;7(2):e000288.
53. Choudhury A, et al. Can we improve the prescribing and delivery of oxygen on a respiratory ward in accordance with new British Thoracic Society oxygen guidelines? BMJ Open Qual. 2018;7(4):e000371.
54. Myers H, et al. Doctors learn new tricks, but do they remember them? Lack of effect of an educational intervention in improving oxygen prescribing. Respirology. 2015;20(8):1229–32.
55. Wilson DF. Oxidative phosphorylation: regulation and role in cellular and tissue metabolism. J Physiol. 2017;595(23):7023–38.
56. Bender DA, Mayes PA. In: DA BKB, Weil PA, Kennelly PJ, Murray RK, Rodwell VW, editors. *Glycolysis & the Oxidation of Pyruvate*, in *Harper's Illustrated Biochemistry*. New York: McGraw-Hill; 2011.
57. Dickinson BC, Chang CJ. Chemistry and biology of reactive oxygen species in signaling or stress responses. Nat Chem Biol. 2011;7(8):504–11.
58. Freeman BA, Crapo JD. Biology of disease: free radicals and tissue injury. Lab Investig. 1982;47(5):412–26.
59. Halliwell B, Gutteridge JM. Oxygen toxicity, oxygen radicals, transition metals and disease. Biochem J. 1984;219(1):1–14.
60. Valko M, et al. Redox- and non-redox-metal-induced formation of free radicals and their role in human disease. Arch Toxicol. 2016;90(1):1–37.
61. Di Meo S, et al. Role of ROS and RNS sources in physiological and pathological conditions. Oxidative Med Cell Longev. 2016;2016:1245049.
62. Rhee SG. Cell signaling. H2O2, a necessary evil for cell signaling. Science. 2006;312(5782):1882–3.
63. Lane N. Oxygen: the molecule that made the world. Oxford: OUP; 2002.
64. Carreau A, et al. Why is the partial oxygen pressure of human tissues a crucial parameter? Small molecules and hypoxia. J Cell Mol Med. 2011;15(6):1239–53.

65. Hafner S, et al. Hyperoxia in intensive care, emergency, and peri-operative medicine: Dr. Jekyll or Mr. Hyde? A 2015 update. Ann Intensive Care. 2015;5(1):42.
66. Jamieson D, et al. The relation of free radical production to hyperoxia. Annu Rev Physiol. 1986;48:703–19.
67. Severinghaus JW, Astrup PB. History of blood gas analysis. IV. Leland Clark's oxygen electrode. J Clin Monit. 1986;2(2):125–39.
68. Glansdorff N, Xu Y, Labedan B. The last universal common ancestor: emergence, constitution and genetic legacy of an elusive forerunner. Biol Direct. 2008;3:29.
69. Ouzounis CA, et al. A minimal estimate for the gene content of the last universal common ancestor--exobiology from a terrestrial perspective. Res Microbiol. 2006;157(1): 57–68.
70. Woese C. The universal ancestor. Proc Natl Acad Sci U S A. 1998;95(12):6854–9.
71. Klotz MG, Loewen PC. The molecular evolution of catalatic hydroperoxidases: evidence for multiple lateral transfer of genes between prokaryota and from bacteria into eukaryota. Mol Biol Evol. 2003;20(7):1098–112.
72. Gerschman R, et al. Oxygen poisoning and x-irradiation: a mechanism in common. Science. 1954;119(3097):623–6.
73. Grocott MP, et al. Arterial blood gases and oxygen content in climbers on Mount Everest. N Engl J Med. 2009;360(2):140–9.
74. Robson AG, Hartung TK, Innes JA. Laboratory assessment of fitness to fly in patients with lung disease: a practical approach. Eur Respir J. 2000;16(2):214–9.
75. Slutsky AS, Rebuck AS. Heart rate response to isocapnic hypoxia in conscious man. Am J Phys. 1978;234(2):H129–32.
76. Easton PA, Slykerman LJ, Anthonisen NR. Ventilatory response to sustained hypoxia in normal adults. J Appl Physiol (1985). 1986;61(3):906–11.
77. Bradley CA, Fleetham JA, Anthonisen NR. Ventilatory control in patients with hypoxemia due to obstructive lung disease. Am Rev Respir Dis. 1979;120(1):21–30.
78. Kogure K, et al. Mechanisms of cerebral vasodilatation in hypoxia. J Appl Physiol. 1970;29(2):223–9.
79. West JW, Guzman SV. Coronary dilatation and constriction visualized by selective arteriography. Circ Res. 1959;7(4):527–36.
80. Weir EK, et al. Acute oxygen-sensing mechanisms. N Engl J Med. 2005;353(19):2042–55.
81. Galatius-Jensen S, et al. Nocturnal hypoxaemia after myocardial infarction: association with nocturnal myocardial ischaemia and arrhythmias. Br Heart J. 1994;72(1):23–30.
82. Gill NP, Wright B, Reilly CS. Relationship between hypoxaemic and cardiac ischaemic events in the perioperative period. Br J Anaesth. 1992;68(5):471–3.
83. Vincent JL, De Backer D. Circulatory shock. N Engl J Med. 2013;369(18):1726–34.
84. Helmerhorst HJ, et al. Metrics of arterial Hyperoxia and associated outcomes in critical care. Crit Care Med. 2017;45(2):187–95.
85. Kilgannon JH, et al. Association between arterial hyperoxia following resuscitation from cardiac arrest and in-hospital mortality. JAMA. 2010;303(21):2165–71.
86. Page D, et al. Emergency department hyperoxia is associated with increased mortality in mechanically ventilated patients: a cohort study. Crit Care. 2018;22(1):9.
87. Lorrain Smith J. The pathological effects due to increase of oxygen tension in the air breathed. J Physiol. 1899;24(1):19–35.
88. Clark JM, Lambertsen CJ. Pulmonary oxygen toxicity: a review. Pharmacol Rev. 1971;23(2):37–133.
89. Kallet RH, Matthay MA. Hyperoxic acute lung injury. Respir Care. 2013;58(1):123–41.
90. Kim V, et al. Oxygen therapy in chronic obstructive pulmonary disease. Proc Am Thorac Soc. 2008;5(4):513–8.
91. Selinger SR, et al. Effects of removing oxygen from patients with chronic obstructive pulmonary disease. Am Rev Respir Dis. 1987;136(1):85–91.
92. Barach AL. Therapeutic use of oxygen in heart disease. Ann Intern Med. 1931;5(10):428.
93. Donald K. Neurological effects of oxygen. Lancet. 1949;257:1056–7.

94. Baldwin ED, Cournand A, Richards DW Jr. Pulmonary insufficiency; a study of 122 cases of chronic pulmonary emphysema. Medicine (Baltimore). 1949;28(2):201–37.
95. Fishman AP, Samet P, Cournand A. Ventilatory drive in chronic pulmonary emphysema. Am J Med. 1955;19(4):533–48.
96. Aubier M, et al. Central respiratory drive in acute respiratory failure of patients with chronic obstructive pulmonary disease. Am Rev Respir Dis. 1980;122(2):191–9.
97. Mithoefer JC, Karetzky MS, Mead GD. Oxygen therapy in respiratory failure. N Engl J Med. 1967;277(18):947–9.
98. Robinson TD, et al. The role of hypoventilation and ventilation-perfusion redistribution in oxygen-induced hypercapnia during acute exacerbations of chronic obstructive pulmonary disease. Am J Respir Crit Care Med. 2000;161(5):1524–9.
99. Sassoon CS, Hassell KT, Mahutte CK. Hyperoxic-induced hypercapnia in stable chronic obstructive pulmonary disease. Am Rev Respir Dis. 1987;135(4):907–11.
100. Campbell EJ, The J. Burns Amberson lecture. The management of acute respiratory failure in chronic bronchitis and emphysema. Am Rev Respir Dis. 1967;96(4):626–39.
101. Rudolf M, Banks RA, Semple SJ. Hypercapnia during oxygen therapy in acute exacerbations of chronic respiratory failure. *Hypothesis revisited.* Lancet. 1977;2(8036):483–6.
102. Ringbaek T, Martinez G, Lange P. The long-term effect of ambulatory oxygen in normoxaemic COPD patients: a randomised study. Chron Respir Dis. 2013;10(2):77–84.
103. Plywaczewski R, et al. Incidence of nocturnal desaturation while breathing oxygen in COPD patients undergoing long-term oxygen therapy. Chest. 2000;117(3):679–83.
104. Sliwinski P, et al. The adequacy of oxygenation in COPD patients undergoing long-term oxygen therapy assessed by pulse oximetry at home. Eur Respir J. 1994;7(2):274–8.
105. Soguel Schenkel N, et al. Oxygen saturation during daily activities in chronic obstructive pulmonary disease. Eur Respir J. 1996;9(12):2584–9.
106. Plant PK, Owen JL, Elliott MW. One year period prevalence study of respiratory acidosis in acute exacerbations of COPD: implications for the provision of non-invasive ventilation and oxygen administration. Thorax. 2000;55(7):550–4.
107. Cameron L, et al. The risk of serious adverse outcomes associated with hypoxaemia and hyperoxaemia in acute exacerbations of COPD. Postgrad Med J. 2012;88(1046):684–9.
108. Roberts CM, et al. Acidosis, non-invasive ventilation and mortality in hospitalised COPD exacerbations. Thorax. 2011;66(1):43–8.
109. Gunawardena KA, et al. Oxygen as a driving gas for nebulisers: safe or dangerous? Br Med J (Clin Res Ed). 1984;288(6413):272–4.
110. Edwards L, et al. Randomised controlled crossover trial of the effect on PtCO2 of oxygen-driven versus air-driven nebulisers in severe chronic obstructive pulmonary disease. Emerg Med J. 2012;29(11):894–8.
111. Bardsley G, et al. Oxygen versus air-driven nebulisers for exacerbations of chronic obstructive pulmonary disease: a randomised controlled trial. BMC Pulm Med. 2018;18(1):157.
112. Kohler E, et al. Lung deposition in cystic fibrosis patients using an ultrasonic or a jet nebulizer. J Aerosol Med. 2003;16(1):37–46.
113. Sepehrvand N, Ezekowitz JA. Oxygen therapy in patients with acute heart failure: friend or foe? JACC Heart Fail. 2016;4(10):783–90.
114. McNulty PH, et al. Effects of supplemental oxygen administration on coronary blood flow in patients undergoing cardiac catheterization. Am J Physiol Heart Circ Physiol. 2005;288(3):H1057–62.
115. Farquhar H, et al. Systematic review of studies of the effect of hyperoxia on coronary blood flow. Am Heart J. 2009;158(3):371–7.
116. Stub D, et al. Air versus oxygen in ST-segment-elevation myocardial infarction. Circulation. 2015;131(24):2143–50.
117. Fonnes S, et al. Perioperative hyperoxia - long-term impact on cardiovascular complications after abdominal surgery, a post hoc analysis of the PROXI trial. Int J Cardiol. 2016;215:238–43.

118. Meyhoff CS, et al. Effect of high perioperative oxygen fraction on surgical site infection and pulmonary complications after abdominal surgery: the PROXI randomized clinical trial. JAMA. 2009;302(14):1543–50.

119. Hofmann R, et al. Oxygen therapy in suspected acute myocardial infarction. N Engl J Med. 2017;377(13):1240–49.

120. Winslow RM. Oxygen: the poison is in the dose. Transfusion. 2013;53(2):424–37.

121. Ihnken K, et al. Normoxic cardiopulmonary bypass reduces oxidative myocardial damage and nitric oxide during cardiac operations in the adult. J Thorac Cardiovasc Surg. 1998;116(2):327–34.

122. Inoue T, et al. Cardioprotective effects of lowering oxygen tension after aortic unclamping on cardiopulmonary bypass during coronary artery bypass grafting. Circ J. 2002;66(8): 718–22.

123. Sparv D, et al. The analgesic effect of oxygen in suspected acute myocardial infarction: a substudy of the DETO2X-AMI trial. JACC Cardiovasc Interv. 2018;11(16):1590–7.

124. Kline KP, Conti CR, Winchester DE. Historical perspective and contemporary management of acute coronary syndromes: from MONA to THROMBINS2. Postgrad Med. 2015;127(8):855–62.

125. Ibanez B, et al. 2017 ESC guidelines for the management of acute myocardial infarction in patients presenting with ST-segment elevation: The Task Force for the management of acute myocardial infarction in patients presenting with ST-segment elevation of the European Society of Cardiology (ESC). Eur Heart J. 2018;39(2):119–77.

126. Bert, P., *La Pression Barométrique*. Recherches de Physiologie Expérimentale. 1878, Paris. 1168.

127. Haldane JBS. *On being one's own rabbit*, in *Possible worlds and other essays*. London: Chatto and Windus; 1927. p. 107–19.

128. Asfar P, et al. Hyperoxia and hypertonic saline in patients with septic shock (HYPERS2S): a two-by-two factorial, multicentre, randomised, clinical trial. Lancet Respir Med. 2017;5(3): 180–90.

129. Floyd TF, et al. Independent cerebral vasoconstrictive effects of hyperoxia and accompanying arterial hypocapnia at 1 ATA. J Appl Physiol. 2003;95(6):2453–61.

130. Floyd TF, et al. Integrity of the cerebral blood-flow response to hyperoxia after cardiopulmonary bypass. J Cardiothorac Vasc Anesth. 2007;21(2):212–7.

131. Ferguson ND. Oxygen in the ICU: too much of a good thing? JAMA. 2016;316(15):1553–4.

132. Damiani E, et al. Arterial hyperoxia and mortality in critically ill patients: a systematic review and meta-analysis. Crit Care. 2014;18(6):711.

133. Vincent JL, Taccone FS, He X. Harmful effects of hyperoxia in postcardiac arrest, sepsis, traumatic brain injury, or stroke: the importance of individualized oxygen therapy in critically ill patients. Can Respir J. 2017;2017:2834956.

134. Dery R, et al. Alveolar collapse induced by denitrogenation. Can Anaesth Soc J. 1965;12(6): 531–57.

135. Rothen HU, et al. Prevention of atelectasis during general anaesthesia. Lancet. 1995; 345(8962):1387–91.

136. Edmark L, et al. Optimal oxygen concentration during induction of general anesthesia. Anesthesiology. 2003;98(1):28–33.

137. Aboab J, et al. Effect of inspired oxygen fraction on alveolar derecruitment in acute respiratory distress syndrome. Intensive Care Med. 2006;32(12):1979–86.

138. Koksal GM, et al. Hyperoxic oxidative stress during abdominal surgery: a randomized trial. J Anesth. 2016;30(4):610–9.

139. de Jonge E, et al. Association between administered oxygen, arterial partial oxygen pressure and mortality in mechanically ventilated intensive care unit patients. Crit Care. 2008;12(6):R156.

140. Palmer E, et al. The association between supra-physiologic arterial oxygen levels and mortality in critically ill patients: a multi-centre observational cohort study. Am J Respir Crit Care Med. 2019;200:1373.

141. Van den Boom W, et al. The search for optimal oxygen saturation targets in critically ill patients. Observational data from large ICU databases. Chest. 2020;157(3):566–73.
142. Investigators I-R, et al. Conservative oxygen therapy during mechanical ventilation in the ICU. N Engl J Med. 2020;382(11):989–98.
143. Schjorring OL, et al. Lower or higher oxygenation targets for acute hypoxemic respiratory failure. N Engl J Med. 2021;384(14):1301–11.
144. Barbateskovic M, et al. Higher vs lower oxygenation strategies in acutely ill adults: a systematic review with meta-analysis and trial sequential analysis. Chest. 2021;159(1):154–73.
145. Hellstrom A, Smith LE, Dammann O. Retinopathy of prematurity. Lancet. 2013;382(9902): 1445–57.
146. Reich B, et al. Hyperoxia and the immature brain. Dev Neurosci. 2017;38:311.
147. Ashton N. Oxygen and the growth and development of retinal vessels. In vivo and in vitro studies. The XX Francis I. Proctor lecture. Am J Ophthalmol. 1966;62(3):412–35.
148. Leigh JM. The evolution of oxygen therapy apparatus. Anaesthesia. 1974;29(4):462–85.
149. Petty TL. Historical highlights of long-term oxygen therapy. Respir Care. 2000;45(1):29–36. discussion 36-8
150. Stark RD, Bishop JM. New method for oxygen therapy in the home using an oxygen concentrator. Br Med J. 1973;2(5858):105–6.
151. Chanques G, et al. Discomfort associated with underhumidified high-flow oxygen therapy in critically ill patients. Intensive Care Med. 2009;35(6):996–1003.
152. Lellouche F, et al. Water content of delivered gases during non-invasive ventilation in healthy subjects. Intensive Care Med. 2009;35(6):987–95.
153. Dawson JA, et al. Quantifying temperature and relative humidity of medical gases used for newborn resuscitation. J Paediatr Child Health. 2014;50(1):24–6.
154. AARC Clinical Practice Guideline. Oxygen therapy for adults in the acute care facility—2002 revision & update. Respir Care. 2002;47(6):717–20.
155. AARC Clinical Practice Guideline. Oxygen therapy in the home or alternate site health care facility—2007 revision & update. Respir Care. 2007;52(1):1063–8.
156. L'Her E, et al. Physiologic effects of noninvasive ventilation during acute lung injury. Am J Respir Crit Care Med. 2005;172(9):1112–8.
157. Campbell EJ, Baker MD, Crites-Silver P. Subjective effects of humidification of oxygen for delivery by nasal cannula. A prospective study. Chest. 1988;93(2):289–93.
158. Franchini ML, et al. Oxygen with cold bubble humidification is no better than dry oxygen in preventing mucus dehydration, decreased mucociliary clearance, and decline in pulmonary function. Chest. 2016;150(2):407–14.
159. Poiroux L, et al. Effect on comfort of administering bubble-humidified or dry oxygen: the Oxyrea non-inferiority randomized study. Ann Intensive Care. 2018;8(1):126.
160. Barach AL. The administration of oxygen by the nasal catheter. JAMA. 1929;93(20):1550–1.
161. Lamb K, Piper D. Southmedic OxyMask(TM) compared with the Hudson RCI((R)) non-rebreather mask(TM): safety and performance comparison. Can J Respir Ther. 2016;52(1): 13–5.
162. Campbell EJ. A method of controlled oxygen administration which reduces the risk of carbon-dioxide retention. Lancet. 1960;2(7140):12–4.
163. Kory RC, et al. Comparative evaluation of oxygen therapy techniques. JAMA. 1962;179: 767–72.
164. Green ID. Choice of method for administration of oxygen. Br Med J. 1967;3(5565):593–6.
165. Poulton TJ, Comer PB, Gibson RL. Tracheal oxygen concentrations with a nasal cannula during oral and nasal breathing. Respir Care. 1980;25(7):739–41.
166. Dunlevy CL, Tyl SE. The effect of oral versus nasal breathing on oxygen concentrations received from nasal cannulas. Respir Care. 1992;37(4):357–60.
167. Wettstein RB, Shelledy DC, Peters JI. Delivered oxygen concentrations using low-flow and high-flow nasal cannulas. Respir Care. 2005;50(5):604–9.
168. MacIntyre NR, Galvin WF, and Mishoe SC. Respiratory care: principles and practice. 2015: Jones & Bartlett Learning.

169. Excellence, N.I.o.H.a.C. Acutely ill patients in hospital: recognition of and response to acute illness in adults in hospital. In: National Institute of health and clinical excellence., N.C. Guideline, Editor. London, England; 2007.

170. Bickler PE, Feiner JR, Severinghaus JW. Effects of skin pigmentation on pulse oximeter accuracy at low saturation. Anesthesiology. 2005;102(4):715–9.

171. Feiner JR, Severinghaus JW, Bickler PE. Dark skin decreases the accuracy of pulse oximeters at low oxygen saturation: the effects of oximeter probe type and gender. Anesth Analg. 2007;105(6 Suppl):S18–23.

172. Louie A, et al. Four types of pulse oximeters accurately detect hypoxia during low perfusion and motion. Anesthesiology. 2018;128(3):520–30.

173. Foglia EE, et al. The effect of skin pigmentation on the accuracy of pulse oximetry in infants with hypoxemia. J Pediatr. 2017;182:375–7. e2

174. Richards NM, Giuliano KK, Jones PG. A prospective comparison of 3 new-generation pulse oximetry devices during ambulation after open heart surgery. Respir Care. 2006;51(1): 29–35.

175. Ross PA, Newth CJ, Khemani RG. Accuracy of pulse oximetry in children. Pediatrics. 2014;133(1):22–9.

176. Singh AK, et al. Comparative evaluation of accuracy of pulse oximeters and factors affecting their performance in a tertiary intensive care unit. J Clin Diagn Res. 2017;11(6):OC05–8.

177. Long term domiciliary oxygen therapy in chronic hypoxic cor pulmonale complicating chronic bronchitis and emphysema. Report of the Medical Research Council Working Party. Lancet. 1981;1(8222):681–6.

178. Dar K, et al. Arterial versus capillary sampling for analysing blood gas pressures. BMJ. 1995;310(6971):24–5.

179. Zavorsky GS, et al. Arterial versus capillary blood gases: a meta-analysis. Respir Physiol Neurobiol. 2007;155(3):268–79.

180. Jubran A. Pulse oximetry. Crit Care. 2015;19:272.

181. Sauty A, et al. Differences in PO2 and PCO2 between arterial and arterialized earlobe samples. Eur Respir J. 1996;9(2):186–9.

182. Jubran A, Tobin MJ. Reliability of pulse oximetry in titrating supplemental oxygen therapy in ventilator-dependent patients. Chest. 1990;97(6):1420–5.

183. Yamamoto LG, et al. Nail polish does not significantly affect pulse oximetry measurements in mildly hypoxic subjects. Respir Care. 2008;53(11):1470–4.

184. Sutcu Cicek H, et al. Effect of nail polish and henna on oxygen saturation determined by pulse oximetry in healthy young adult females. Emerg Med J. 2011;28(9):783–5.

185. Alam N, et al. The impact of the use of the Early Warning Score (EWS) on patient outcomes: a systematic review. Resuscitation. 2014;85(5):587–94.

186. Churpek MM, et al. Derivation of a cardiac arrest prediction model using ward vital signs*. Crit Care Med. 2012;40(7):2102–8.

187. Jo S, et al. Predictive value of the National Early Warning Score-Lactate for mortality and the need for critical care among general emergency department patients. J Crit Care. 2016;36:60–8.

188. Jansen JO, Cuthbertson BH. Detecting critical illness outside the ICU: the role of track and trigger systems. Curr Opin Crit Care. 2010;16(3):184–90.

189. Smith GB, et al. The ability of the National Early Warning Score (NEWS) to discriminate patients at risk of early cardiac arrest, unanticipated intensive care unit admission, and death. Resuscitation. 2013;84(4):465–70.

190. Churpek MM, Adhikari R, Edelson DP. The value of vital sign trends for detecting clinical deterioration on the wards. Resuscitation. 2016;102:1–5.

191. Gao H, et al. Systematic review and evaluation of physiological track and trigger warning systems for identifying at-risk patients on the ward. Intensive Care Med. 2007;33(4): 667–79.

192. Smith ME, et al. Early warning system scores for clinical deterioration in hospitalized patients: a systematic review. Ann Am Thorac Soc. 2014;11(9):1454–65.

193. Churpek MM, et al. Quick sepsis-related organ failure assessment, systemic inflammatory response syndrome, and early warning scores for detecting clinical deterioration in infected patients outside the intensive care unit. Am J Respir Crit Care Med. 2017;195(7):906–11.

194. Usman OA, Usman AA, Ward MA. Comparison of SIRS, qSOFA, and NEWS for the early identification of sepsis in the Emergency Department. Am J Emerg Med. 2018;37:1490.

195. Sutherasan Y, et al. The impact of introducing the early warning scoring system and protocol on clinical outcomes in tertiary referral university hospital. Ther Clin Risk Manag. 2018;14:2089–95.

196. McNeill G, Bryden D. Do either early warning systems or emergency response teams improve hospital patient survival? A systematic review. Resuscitation. 2013;84:1652–67.

197. Kivipuro M, et al. National early warning score (NEWS) in a Finnish multidisciplinary emergency department and direct vs. late admission to intensive care. Resuscitation. 2018;128:164–9.

198. Schein RM, et al. Clinical antecedents to in-hospital cardiopulmonary arrest. Chest. 1990;98(6):1388–92.

199. Churpek MM, et al. Predicting cardiac arrest on the wards: a nested case-control study. Chest. 2012;141(5):1170–6.

200. Ludikhuize J, et al. Identification of deteriorating patients on general wards; measurement of vital parameters and potential effectiveness of the Modified Early Warning Score. J Crit Care. 2012;27(4):424. e7-13

201. Galhotra S, et al. Mature rapid response system and potentially avoidable cardiopulmonary arrests in hospital. Qual Saf Health Care. 2007;16(4):260–5.

202. Kwack WG, et al. Evaluation of the SpO2/FiO2 ratio as a predictor of intensive care unit transfers in respiratory ward patients for whom the rapid response system has been activated. PLoS One. 2018;13(7):e0201632.

203. Lellouche F, L'Her E. Usual and advanced monitoring in patients receiving oxygen therapy. Respir Care. 2020;65(10):1591–600.

204. Viglino D, et al. Evaluation of a new respiratory monitoring tool "Early Warning ScoreO2" for patients admitted at the emergency department with dyspnea. Resuscitation. 2020;148:59–65.

205. Hess DR. et al. Respiratory care: principles and practice. 2012: Jones & Bartlett Learning.

206. Neu M. Ein Verfahren zur Stickoxydulsauerstoffnarkose. Munch Med Wochenschr. 1910;57:1873–5.

207. Lenfant C. Shattuck lecture—clinical research to clinical practice—lost in translation? N Engl J Med. 2003;349(9):868–74.

208. Scales DC, Adhikari NK. Lost in (knowledge) translation: "all breakthrough, no follow through"? Crit Care Med. 2008;36(5):1654–5.

209. BR., O.D. British Thoracic Society. Emergency oxygen audit 2013. . audit-and-quality-improvement/audit-reports/bts-emergency-oxygen-audit-report-2013 2013 January 15, 2019]; https://www.brit-thoracic.org.uk/document-library/audit-and-quality-improvement/audit-reports/bts-emergency-oxygen-audit-report-2013/.

210. Pretto JJ, et al. Multicentre audit of inpatient management of acute exacerbations of chronic obstructive pulmonary disease: comparison with clinical guidelines. Intern Med J. 2012;42(4):380–7.

211. Roberts CM, et al. European hospital adherence to GOLD recommendations for chronic obstructive pulmonary disease (COPD) exacerbation admissions. Thorax. 2013;68(12):1169–71.

212. Dojat M, Brochard L. Knowledge-based systems for automatic ventilatory management. Respir Care Clin N Am. 2001;7(3):379–96. viii

213. Lellouche F, et al. A multicenter randomized trial of computer-driven protocolized weaning from mechanical ventilation. Am J Respir Crit Care Med. 2006;174(8):894–900.

214. Arnal JM, et al. Automatic selection of breathing pattern using adaptive support ventilation. Intensive Care Med. 2008;34(1):75–81.

215. Lellouche F, et al. Evaluation of fully automated ventilation: a randomized controlled study in post-cardiac surgery patients. Intensive Care Med. 2013;39(3):463–71.

216. Bouchard PA, et al. Closed-loop oxygen titration system (FreeO2) during NIV in healthy subjects with induced hypoxemia. Am J Respir Crit Care Med. 2012;185:A6492.
217. Lellouche F, et al. Automatic oxygen titration during walking in subjects with COPD: a randomized crossover controlled study. Respir Care. 2016;61(11):1456–64.
218. Vivodtzev I, et al. Automated O2 titration improves exercise capacity in patients with hypercapnic chronic obstructive pulmonary disease: a randomised controlled cross-over trial. Thorax. 2019;74(3):298–301.
219. Lellouche F, et al. Automated oxygen titration and weaning with FreeO2 in patients with acute exacerbation of COPD: a pilot randomized trial. Int J Chron Obstruct Pulmon Dis. 2016;11:1983–90.
220. L'Her E, et al. Automatic versus manual oxygen administration in the emergency department. Eur Respir J. 2017;50:1.
221. Lellouche F, et al. Evaluation of automated oxygen flowrate titration (FreeO2) in a model of induced cyclic desaturations in healthy subjects reproducing desaturations during central Apneas. Am J Respir Crit Care Med. 2017;195:A2585.
222. Dupin C, et al. Automatic oxygen titration improves exercise tolerance in patients with idiopathic lung fibrosis. Am J Respir Crit Care Med. 2018;197:A4268.
223. Huynh-Ky M. et al. *Closed-loop adjustment of oxygen flowrate with FreeO2 in patients with acute coronary syndrome: comparison of two SpO2 target and manual adjustment. A randomized controlled study.* Annals of Intensive Care, 2017.
224. Roué JM. et al. *Automatic oxygen flow titration in spontaneously breathing children: An open-label randomized controlled pilot study.* Pediatric Pulmonol. 2020;55(11):3180–88.
225. Lellouche F, et al. Automated oxygen titration and weaning with FreeO2 during acute exacerbation of COPD. Am J Respir Crit Care Med. 2018;197:A4555.
226. L'Her E, et al. Automated oxygen administration versus conventional oxygen therapy after major abdominal or thoracic surgery: study protocol for an international multicentre randomised controlled study. BMJ Open. 2019;9(1):e023833.
227. L'Her E, et al. Automated closed-loop versus standard manual oxygen administration after major abdominal or thoracic surgery: an international multicentre randomised controlled study. Eur Respir J. 2021;57(1):2000182.
228. Poder TG, et al. Cost-effectiveness of FreeO2 in patients with chronic obstructive pulmonary disease hospitalised for acute exacerbations: analysis of a pilot study in Quebec. BMJ Open. 2018;8(1):e018835.
229. Ouanes I, et al. Automatic oxygen administration and weaning in patients following mechanical ventilation. J Crit Care. 2020;61:45–51.
230. Bourassa S, et al. Oxygen conservation methods with automated titration. Respir Care. 2020;65:1433.
231. Denault MH, et al. Automatic versus manual oxygen titration in patients requiring supplemental oxygen in the hospital: a systematic review and meta-analysis. Respiration. 2019;98(2):178–188.
232. Hansen EF, et al. Automatic oxygen titration with O2matic(R) to patients admitted with COVID-19 and hypoxemic respiratory failure. Eur Clin Respir J. 2020;7(1):1833695.
233. Dunne PJ, McCoy RW. Patient-centric LTOT: no room for complacency. Respir Care. 2011;56(4):536–7.
234. Winck JC. Intelligent oxygen delivery in the acute setting: "Don't think twice, it's all right". Eur Respir J. 2017;50:1.
235. Lellouche F, Lipes J, L'Her E. Optimal oxygen titration in patients with chronic obstructive pulmonary disease: a role for automated oxygen delivery? Can Respir J. 2013;20(4):259–61.
236. Vincent JL. No room for hyperoxia or hypertonic saline in septic shock. Lancet Respir Med. 2017;5(3):158–9.

High-Flow Nasal Cannula: Technical Aspects in Adults and Children

2

Amanda Corley, Donna Franklin, Andreas Schibler, and John F. Fraser

2.1 Components of High-Flow Nasal Cannula Delivery System

The system used to deliver oxygen therapy through high-flow nasal cannulae (HFNC) consists of four components: a gas blender and flow meter; an active humidifier; a heated inspiratory circuit; and the nasal cannula interface (see Fig. 2.1).

2.1.1 Gas Flow and FiO_2 Delivery

In contrast to standard oxygen delivery devices, gas flow rate and FiO_2 can be adjusted independently of each other. Commercially available HFNC systems have the capability to deliver flow rates between 2 and 100 L/min [1–4]. Commonly used flow rates for neonatal, paediatric and adult patients are detailed in Table 2.1. Depending on the HFNC delivery system applied, medical gases are attached to the device or, alternatively, air is entrained using a turbine and supplemental oxygen is added. An air/oxygen blender can deliver an FiO_2 of between 0.21 and 1.0 and can be either integrated within or attached to the delivery system.

An advantage of the HFNC system over standard oxygen therapy is its ability to more adequately meet, and indeed exceed, the inspiratory demands of the patient with higher inspiratory flows, providing a more accurately delivered FiO_2 and

A. Corley (✉) · J. F. Fraser
Critical Care Research Group, The Prince Charles Hospital and University of Queensland, Brisbane, QLD, Australia
e-mail: amanda.corley@health.qld.gov.au; j.fraser@uq.edu.au

D. Franklin · A. Schibler
Paediatric Critical Care Research Group, Queensland Children's Hospital and The University of Queensland, Brisbane, QLD, Australia
e-mail: d.franklin2@uq.edu.au; a.schibler@uq.edu.au

© Springer Nature Switzerland AG 2021
A. Carlucci, S. M. Maggiore (eds.), *High Flow Nasal Cannula*,
https://doi.org/10.1007/978-3-030-42454-1_2

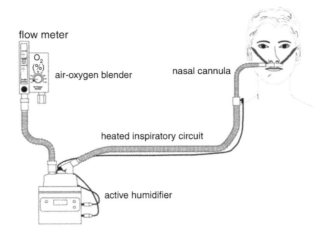

Fig. 2.1 Components of a high-flow nasal cannula delivery system. The air/oxygen blender and flow meter allow the delivery of a FiO$_2$ between 0.21 and 1.0 at a flow of up to 60 L/min. An active humidifier heats the gas which is then delivered by a heated inspiratory limb to the nasal cannula. (From Laurent Papazian L, et al. Use of high-flow nasal cannula oxygenation in ICU adults: a narrative review. Intensive Care Medicine 2016:42(4) DOI https://doi.org/10.1007/s00134-016-4277-8 (used with permission))

Table 2.1 Flow rates routinely prescribed for high-flow therapy. Source: Children's Health Queensland Hospital and Health Service. Guideline: nasal high flow therapy—management of the paediatric patient receiving high flow therapy. 2019. Queensland Government Department of Health, Brisbane

Weight	Flow rates
Neonates	Up to 8 L/min
0–12 kg	2 L/kg/min up to maximum of 25 L/min
13–15 kg	2 L/kg/min up to maximum of 30 L/min
16–30 kg	35–40 L/min
31–50 kg	40–50 L/min
>50 kg (adults)	40–70 L/min

reducing inspiratory resistance [5, 6]. Inspiratory flow demands of adult patients with acute respiratory failure can range from 30 L/min to more than 120 L/min [7]. Therefore, when the patient is supported by standard low-flow oxygen (i.e., at a flow of up to 15 L/min), the difference between delivered flow and inspiratory flow is large. This results in entrainment of room air, significantly lowering delivered FiO$_2$ [8]. The ability of HFNC to deliver flows of up to 70 L/min (depending on the type of device used) means that the increased flow demands are more adequately matched, providing a more reliable FiO$_2$. It must be noted however that the delivered FiO$_2$ in patients whose inspiratory flow demands exceed 70 L/min will ultimately be diluted by entrained room air. In a study of healthy volunteers [9], increased inspiratory demand was simulated by exercise to achieve a peak inspiratory flow rate of >100 L/min. Higher peak flows were associated with lower delivered FiO_2 compared with FiO_2 delivered to resting subjects, indicating room air entrainment [9].

The estimated positive airway pressure using 2 L/kg/min in infants <12 months of age is approximately 4–6 cmH_2O [10]. Observational clinical scoring systems allow the clinician to monitor and track the severity of the patient's work of breathing; however this has its limitations as it is subjective and based on the clinician's level of experience [11]. HFNC flow rates delivered according to Table 2.1 for children will exceed the patient's inspiratory demands, offload the diaphragm and generate moderate inspiratory support and positive expiratory pressures, thereby significantly reducing work of breathing and improving gas exchange [12]. Using appropriate flows as shown in Table 2.1 can reduce the need for escalation of respiratory support. However, if FiO_2 is greater than 60% to achieve clinically acceptable saturations, escalation of care and management may be required.

The amount of flow delivered to the adult patient is also important due to the beneficial physiological effects it elicits [13–15]. Increasing HFNC flow rates result in linear improvements (increases or decreases as appropriate) in end-expiratory lung volume, oxygenation, respiratory rate and positive airway pressure [13–15]. Exponential decreases in the work of breathing and minute ventilation are also associated with increasing HFNC flows [14].

It is acknowledged when applying HFNC to support the breathing cycle in children that the flow requirement does not increase linearly with weight or growth. The respiratory flow and volume changes during the respiratory cycle follow the growth of the child. At the age of 4 years and older the relative size of the lung and the requirement of respiratory support start to be more equal to an adult; hence the initial 2 L/kg/min of support needs to be adapted accordingly.

2.1.2   Humidification

Adequate humidification is essential to the successful delivery of oxygen therapy via HFNC [2] as high flow of gas without humidification is poorly tolerated. HFNC delivery systems require an active heated humidifier to optimally condition the inspired gas to 37 °C in adults and 34–37 °C in children, with 44 mg H_2O/L. This circumvents problems associated with delivering dry, cold gases, such as bronchoconstriction [16, 17], decreased compliance [18], discomfort [5, 19] and decreased mucociliary clearance [20]. In contrast, delivering adequately warmed and humidified gas improves tolerability and comfort for the patient [5, 19]; facilitates secretion clearance [21]; and reduces metabolic costs associated with gas conditioning usually performed by the nasopharynx [6].

It is crucial that sufficient time is allowed for the humidifier to achieve the required maximum temperature prior to applying HFNC to the patient as this ensures that optimal humidity is delivered from commencement of therapy. Commencing high flows prior to adequate heating and humidifying of the gas results in discomfort and mucosal irritation and ultimately poor patient compliance with the therapy. It is important to note that if flow demands exceed flow delivery, 100% humidity may not be provided to the patient due to the entrainment of room air [22].

2.1.3 Inspiratory Tubing

The warmed humidified gas is delivered to the patient via a single-limb-heated inspiratory circuit. The circuit (or tubing) is lightweight and flexible with a heater wire embedded within the tubing wall and is insulated to minimise condensation and the effects from ambient air temperature. Like all humidified circuits, there is a chance of condensation or 'rain out' occurring which reduces the efficiency of humidification and increases infection risk [23]. Both circuit design and flow influence the amount of condensation; however ambient air temperature is the strongest predictor of condensation forming within the circuit [24, 25]; therefore, where practicable, the inspiratory circuit should be kept away from air-conditioning vents and/or fans to prevent condensate from developing.

2.1.4 Nasal Cannula Interface

The heated, humidified gas is delivered directly into the nostrils via two cannulae which should sit snugly without occluding them completely. In neonates and paediatrics, it is recommended that the cannula-to-nostril diameter ratio should not exceed 0.8 and there is a visible gap between the cannula and the patient's nostril. Many of the available HFNC resemble a somewhat larger low-flow nasal cannula; however two types of cannula have a slightly different design (Comfort Flo Plus, Teleflex, and Optiflow, Fisher & Paykel). These products have wider bore cannulae made of softer silicone; attach to the heated inspiratory circuit with larger diameter corrugated tubing; and have a clip to hold the corrugated tubing and thus minimise cannula displacement from the nostrils. Depending on which commercially available device is used, the nasal cannulae are held in place with a head strap; secured behind the head; or hooked over the ears and secured under the chin. In infants and children, the nasal cannula can be secured to the child's face with adhesive tape of premade Velcro systems, which allows easy removal and replacement when administering bronchodilator medication. When compared with a Venturi mask, Maggiore et al. [26] found that HFNC use resulted in significantly fewer interface dislodgements and the authors purport that improved patient comfort was an important factor in this finding. Interestingly, the study authors also found that patients receiving HFNC therapy had significantly fewer episodes of desaturation than those receiving oxygen via a Venturi mask and attributed this to better therapy tolerance and, therefore, fewer interface displacements. Appropriate cannula size selection is important and should be done in consultation with the manufacturer's recommendations but should also be directed by cannula tolerability and comfort.

2.2   Commercially Available HFNC Devices

Currently, the most widely used HFNC systems are manufactured by Fisher & Paykel Healthcare (Auckland, New Zealand) and Vapotherm (Precision Flow Plus; Vapotherm, Inc., Exeter, NH). Fisher & Paykel products are the AIRVO™ 2 System, consisting of a humidifier with an integrated flow source that entrains room air and to which supplemental oxygen may be added, or a non-integrated system which consists of the humidifier, a gas blender with oxygen analyser and flow meter (Optiflow™ system: Optiflow nasal cannulae, RT-heated delivery tubing and MR850-heated humidifier). Precision Flow Plus by Vapotherm is an integrated HFNC delivery system where the humidification chamber, gas blender and oxygen analyser are incorporated into a single delivery device. Figure 2.2 shows these HFNC delivery systems. Other commercially available HFNC systems include Teleflex Comfort Flo® HFNC Therapy (Morrisville, NC, USA); Flexicare Veoflo® (Mountain Ash, Wales, UK); Armstrong AquaNASE® and NeoFlow (Coleraine, Northern Ireland, UK); and ResMed AcuCare™ (San Diego, CA, USA).

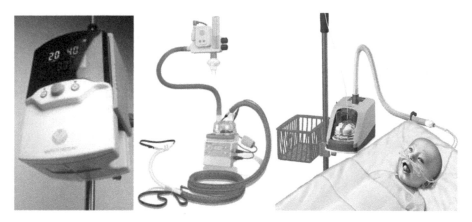

Fig. 2.2 More commonly used HFNC delivery systems. From left to right: Precision Flow (Vapotherm). (From F. Javier Pilar and Yolanda M. Lopez Fernandez. High-Flow Nasal Cannula Oxygen in Acute Respiratory Post-extubation Failure in Pediatric Patients: Key Practical Topics and Clinical Implications In: Esquinas A. (eds). Noninvasive Mechanical Ventilation and Difficult Weaning in Critical Care. Springer, Cham, image used with permission); Optiflow™ system (Fisher & Paykel Healthcare); Optiflow™ Junior with AIRVO 2™ (Fisher & Paykel Healthcare, image used with permission).

2.3 Contraindications and Adverse Events

2.3.1 Contraindications

Given the current lack of consensus guidelines regarding the use of HFNC, guidance regarding contraindications is scarce. Contraindications to HFNC use predominantly focus on airway protection and upper airway abnormalities. Additionally, there are some conditions which warrant careful use of HFNC (Table 2.2).

2.3.2 Adverse Events

Reports of adverse events in the literature are rare. Most adverse events are related to patient discomfort due to either heat or high flow of delivered gas resulting in nasal discomfort or rhinorrhoea. Nagata and colleagues [27] investigated domiciliary use of HFNC and reported minor adverse events, including night sweats, nasal discharge, insomnia, and a skin rash. Gastric distension associated with HFNC use has also been reported [28, 29], in addition to air leaks in neonatal and paediatric population causing barotrauma [30]. There is always the potential for the patient to develop skin or mucosal injuries from the cannula interface so care must be taken to prevent this.

Kang and colleagues [31] found in a retrospective analysis that patients receiving HFNC for greater than 48 h who required subsequent intubation had higher ICU mortality and less extubation success and were more difficult to wean from mechanical ventilation. Similar to delaying intubation with NIV [32, 33], care must be taken to recognise signs of worsening respiratory failure early and escalate supportive measures appropriately. The potential risk of hyperinflation when HFNC are used in

Table 2.2 Conditions for which high-flow nasal cannula is contraindicated or should be used with caution. Adapted from Parke R.L. (2016) High-Flow Nasal Cannula Oxygen in Acute Respiratory Failure After Extubation: Key Practical Topics and Clinical Implications. In: Esquinas A. (eds) Noninvasive Mechanical Ventilation and Difficult Weaning in Critical Care. Springer, Cham

Contraindications to HFNC use	Conditions which warrant careful HFNC use
Unable to protect airway	Severe agitation, unable to follow commands
Life-threatening hypoxia	Respiratory acidosis
Base-of-skull fracture	Swallowing impairment
Maxillofacial trauma	Recent neurosurgery or upper gastrointestinal
Recent upper airway surgery	surgery
Nasal obstruction, e.g. tumour, polyps, septal deformity/trauma	Poor skin integrity of face, e.g. burns
Severe oropharyngeal mucositis	
Foreign-body aspiration	
Epistaxis	
Specific additional contraindications to HFNC use in infants and children	**Specific additional conditions which warrant careful HFNC use in infants and children**
Choanal atresia	Bulbar dysfunction
Certain craniofacial malformations	Neuromuscular hypotonia
Severe central apnoea	
Trans-oesophageal fistula pre- and post-op	

patients with severe obstructive lung disease should be considered if such patients are seen to clinically deteriorate or desaturate on the initiation of HFNC.

2.4 Initiation, Maintenance, and Weaning

2.4.1 Setting for HFNC Delivery and Staffing

2.4.1.1 Adult Considerations

Adults with acute respiratory failure requiring support with HFNC have often failed standard low-flow oxygen therapy so must be considered at higher risk of worsening failure or requiring mechanical ventilation. Therefore, HFNC therapy should be delivered in a setting which is amenable to close monitoring and observation; has appropriately trained staff; and can deal with a deteriorating patient. For these reasons, HFNC therapy for acute respiratory failure may be best delivered in critical care areas or the emergency department. This recommendation is not related to HFNC itself, but rather to the acuity of the patient. Once the patient is requiring a gas flow rate and concentration of oxygen which could be safely managed in a ward environment then transfer to a lower acuity setting could be considered, provided that the patient has been stable for a sustained period of time. Indeed, HFNC have been successfully used in adult ward patients experiencing ongoing mild-to-moderate respiratory failure [34, 35] and in the home for stable chronic lung conditions [27, 36]. If adult patients on HFNC are to be managed in a ward environment, a clear protocol must be in place which articulates the maximal flow rate and FiO_2 safely deliverable in the ward and an escalation plan once that threshold is met.

Whilst the delivery of invasive or non-invasive ventilation dictates a 1:1 or 1:2 nurse:patient ratio, the staffing ratio for a patient receiving HFNC should be determined on a patient acuity basis. For unstable adult patients receiving HFNC for acute respiratory failure, higher nurse-to-patient ratios would be considered safe, for instance 1:2 or 1:3. Once physiological parameters have stabilised on HFNC, then it would be reasonable to reduce the staffing ratio.

2.4.1.2 Paediatric Considerations

In contrast to the adult population, the use of HFNC therapy in infants with bronchiolitis as a primary oxygen therapy or as a rescue therapy once standard oxygen therapy has failed can be recommended for all clinical settings, which include emergency departments, general wards and intensive care [1, 37, 38]. The greatest clinical benefit is the reduction in work of breathing and CO_2 washout. In children with acute respiratory distress, HFNC therapy in general ward settings is very commonly used with great benefit and safety efficacy, which includes children with asthma.

In paediatrics, there is high-grade evidence that 1:4 nurse:patient ratio is safe and effective [1, 37, 38]. Small children and infants can safely be cared for in the emergency department or paediatric ward settings on flows outlined in Table 2.1 with nurse:patient ratio remaining the same as for standard oxygen therapy delivery. It is only when the child deteriorates and requires escalation of care that the nurse:patient ratio or clinical environment is changed to a higher level, such as high dependency or intensive care [1].

2.4.2   Initiation and Maintenance of HFNC Therapy

Due to the lack of efficacy data on optimal HFNC commencement time frames or the way in which it is delivered, there are currently no consensus guidelines regarding initiation, maintenance or weaning of HFNC oxygen therapy. Most data supporting adult use of HFNC derive from trials including patients with undifferentiated hypoxaemic acute respiratory failure, with little attention given to tailored HFNC settings during treatment initiation. Therefore, treatment should be guided by individual patient response to the therapy with consideration of the underlying condition.

In adults, there is no evidence-based starting flow rate for HFNC provided by manufacturers or the literature; however, given that many of the physiological benefits of HFNC therapy are dependent on higher flows [13–15], flow rates for adults should commence at no lower than 40 L/min. Initially, FiO_2 should be commenced at a level appropriate to patient oxygenation status. Flow should then be titrated upwards in 5–10 L/min increments to a target of 60 L/min, using a reduction in respiratory rate and breathing difficulty, and patient comfort as a guide. Additionally, higher flows rates can be expected to reduce entrainment of room air by more adequately matching inspiratory demand [6]. Therefore, oxygenation should improve with increasing flow, and FiO_2 could be titrated downward. If oxygenation does not improve with increased flow, FiO_2 should then be titrated up to reach the desired SpO_2 target [39].

Adult patients often need to 'settle in' to the sensation of the high nasal flow but once established, the therapy is well tolerated. Adequate education regarding the foreign sensation of nasal heat, humidity and flow can assist successful initiation of HFNC therapy. Some patients may need more time than others when adjusting to HFNC and, if their physiological condition permits, slow up-titration of flow can help in this regard.

When caring for adults receiving HFNC, flow rate and FiO_2 settings should be adjusted to the changing condition of the patient. If hypoxia and tachypnoea persist, flow should be increased in 5 L/min increments in the first instance to better meet inspiratory demands rather than increasing FiO_2 [39]. If physiological targets are not met with increased flow, then FiO_2 must be titrated to maintain adequate oxygenation. Close observation for signs of deterioration is crucial (see Section: Predictors of Failure) and escalation of respiratory support should not be delayed as doing so may lead to adverse patient outcomes [31]. In infants and children with increasing hypoxia and persistent tachypnoea, consideration for an increase in flow should occur in a high-dependency or intensive care setting. This includes flows up to 3 L/kg/min for infants less than 12 months of age, and in older children, increasing and maximising the flow as high as the child can tolerate for a clinical benefit to be seen.

In an informative narrative review of HFNC therapy in adults experiencing acute hypoxaemic respiratory failure, Ischaki and colleagues [40] propose a comprehensive evidence-based algorithm to guide HFNC therapy (Fig. 2.3). The authors suggest that if an adult patient presents with hypoxaemic respiratory failure (PaO_2/FiO_2

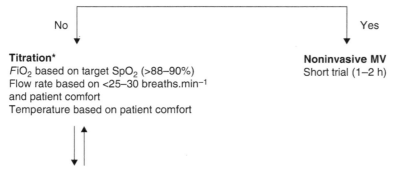

Acute hypoxaemic respiratory failure#
Criteria for immediate or imminent intubation are present
(*i.e.* impaired consciousness and/or persistent shock¶)

No | Yes

NHF initiation
FiO_2 100%, flow rate 60 L·min⁻¹
Temperature 37°C

Intubation and invasive MV
NHF for improving pre-oxygenation
and peri-laryngoscopy oxygenation
FiO_2 100%, flow rate 60 L·min⁻¹

Within
1–2 h

Monitoring
Presence of one of the following: respiratory rate > 35 breaths-min⁻¹, SpO_2 < 88–90%
Theraco-abdominal asynchrony and/or persistent auxiliary muscle use, respiratory acidosis
($PaCO_2$ >45 mmHg with pH < 7.35)

No | Yes

Titration*
FiO_2 based on target SpO_2 (>88–90%)
Flow rate based on <25–30 breaths.min⁻¹
and patient comfort
Temperature based on patient comfort

Noninvasive MV
Short trial (1–2 h)

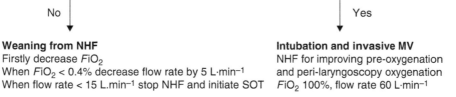

Monitoring
Presence of one of the following within hours (maximum 48 h), besides optimum NHF
titration: respiratory rate >35 breaths.min–1, SpO_2 < 88–90%, thoraco-abdominal
asynchrony and/or persistent auxiliary muscle use, respiratory acidosis ($PaCO_2$ > 45 mmHg
with pH < 7.35), haemodynamic instability§

No | Yes

Weaning from NHF
Firstly decrease FiO_2
When FiO_2 < 0.4% decrease flow rate by 5 L·min⁻¹
When flow rate < 15 L.min⁻¹ stop NHF and initiate SOT

Intubation and invasive MV
NHF for improving pre-oxygenation
and peri-laryngoscopy oxygenation
FiO_2 100%, flow rate 60 L·min⁻¹

Fig. 2.3 Suggested management algorithm for adult patients in acute hypoxaemic respiratory failure. #Arterial oxygen tension (PaO2)/fraction of inspired oxygen (FiO2) ratio < 300; patients with arterial carbon dioxide tension (PaCO2) > 45 mmHg and pH <7.35 are excluded. ¶Systolic arterial blood pressure < 90 mmHg with adequate fluid administration; §haemodynamic instability is defined as a heart rate > 140 beats/min or a change of >20% from baseline and/or a systolic arterial blood pressure of >180 mmHg, <90 mmHg or a decrease of >40 mmHg from baseline; NHF, nasal high-flow oxygen therapy; MV, mechanical ventilation; SOT, standard oxygen therapy. (Reproduced with permission of the © ERS 2019: European Respiratory Review 26 (145) 170028; DOI: https://doi.org/10.1183/16000617.0028-2017 Published 9 August 2017)

ratio < 300) without hypercapnia and acidosis ($PaCO_2$ > 45 mmHg and pH < 7.35) then HFNC can be used as a primary supportive therapy if intubation criteria are not met, or, if intubation criteria are met, as a pre-oxygenation tool during laryngoscopy with maximum settings (flow rate 60 L/min with 100% FiO_2). If the adult patient is not requiring imminent intubation, HFNC should be applied as soon as able at a maximum gas flow rate with optimal humidity to assist in relieving dyspnoea and reduce work of breathing. Continuous monitoring is required to ensure response to therapy, and early and appropriate escalation of treatment should ensue if the desired response to HFNC is not achieved.

Based on previous work from Sztrymf and colleagues on adults [41], the presence of one of $SpO2$ < 88–90%; respiratory rate > 35 breaths per minute; thoracoabdominal asynchrony; or auxiliary use of respiratory muscles early after HFNC initiation may indicate non-response to therapy. Ischaki et al. [40] also advocate short trials of NIV prior to considering intubation if non-response to HFNC is apparent. Importantly, they advise a maximum window of 48 h in which to determine the success of HFNC therapy as evidence shows that delaying intubation beyond this time frame results in adverse patient outcomes [31]. Given that early signs of non-response to HFNC exist and that the patient is closely monitored, appropriate escalation of respiratory support must be attended promptly. Evidence-based guidelines to inform clinical practice in this area are eagerly awaited.

In infants and children, the flow rates as per Table 2.1 are commenced and increased slowly to reach the required set flow rate over 2–3 min to ensure comfort and less distress for the child. If an oxygen requirement is present, FiO_2 is increased slowly to meet the target SpO_2. However, the child may improve on HFNC delivered with room air only and it may be appropriate to commence HFNC on room air only for the first 10 min, only increasing FiO_2 if the target saturations cannot be achieved. In severely unwell children, HFNC can be commenced with a higher FiO_2. The use of FiO_2 > 0.6 is discouraged in children and should only be used as a bridge to NIV or intubation. In infants with bronchiolitis, close observation of heart rate and respiratory rate should be given, and if there is not a 10–20% decrease within the first 1–2 h of high-flow treatment, or if the $FiO2$ increases >40%, then higher level of care should be considered [42].

2.4.3　Monitoring during HFNC

Similar to any therapy commenced in a potentially unstable patient, close monitoring of the patient's clinical condition is important. For unstable patients, at a minimum, continuous oxygen saturation monitoring should occur, and continuous heart rate and respiratory rate monitoring may also be appropriate. Hourly checks of the HFNC circuit must be performed to ensure optimal function. Depending on institutional protocol, arterial blood gas analysis may be useful soon after initiation of therapy to monitor for hypercapnia and acidosis, and thereafter if signs of deterioration in respiratory status are noted.

2.4.4 Weaning

As with other forms of respiratory support, weaning adult patients from the delivered support can safely commence once respiratory parameters are within a predetermined satisfactory range. For adult patients, it is advisable to decrease FiO_2 first, and then decrease flow in increments of 5 L/min until a rate of 20 L/min is achieved. If signs of respiratory distress develop during the weaning process, return to the previous support level. If the patient is stable on 20 L/min, a change to low-flow oxygen is indicated. Refer to algorithm for the management of adult patients in Fig. 2.3 [40].

In infants and children who are administered flows according to Table 2.1, FiO_2 is gradually weaned to room air first and then flow is switched off without further weaning. It is preferential to have the child on room air for 1 h to assess stability, prior to switching off flow and removing the nasal cannula. Should the infant or child further deteriorate or become hypoxic again, treatment is recommenced at the previous flow settings and increase the FiO_2 as required to meet target saturations. A proportion of infants and children may remain stable on HFNC with room air only for their full admission and it is advisable to apply the room air-only HFNC for a minimum of 2 h before turning off the flow.

2.4.5 Predictors of Treatment Failure

In adult patients, a number of important studies have been conducted which give some insight into factors associated with HFNC treatment failure; however more work needs to be conducted in this area to validate or establish predictors of non-response for the many different aetiologies of respiratory failure. Most of the evidence derives from studies where patients were treated with HFNC for undifferentiated hypoxaemic respiratory failure; therefore the utility of these predictors for more specific aetiologies of hypoxaemic respiratory failure is unclear.

Independent predictors of HFNC failure in adults requiring escalation to NIV or intubation include higher severity of illness scores [43–46], specifically a SOFA score of ≥4 and an APACHE II score of ≥12 [47]; concurrent haemodynamic failure and need for vasopressor support [43, 47]; and presence of an extensive pleural effusion [44]. The presence of any of these should alert the treating team that the patient is at high risk of HFNC failure and perhaps should guide them to another course of treatment, such as mechanical ventilation, if appropriate.

Specific physiological signs have been identified as predicting or indicating non-response to HFNC therapy. A decrease in respiratory rate appears to be the most important indicator of HFNC success. Studies in both adults and paediatrics [41, 42, 45, 48] have demonstrated that no reduction in respiratory rate early after HFNC initiation is associated with HFNC failure and subsequent need for escalation of respiratory support. In adults, Sztrymf et al. [41] found that non-response of respiratory rate within 30 min of NHF therapy commencement was an early predictor of subsequent tracheal intubation. Similarly, Frat et al. [48] identified that in 8 of 28 patients who required intubation, a respiratory rate of ≥ 30 breaths/min within the first hour of treatment predicted intubation with a sensitivity of 94.1% and specificity of 87.5%. Thoracoabdominal asynchrony, an indicator of increased work of breathing, has also been identified as an important predictor of NHF failure in adults, with significantly more adult patients requiring intubation if exhibiting this sign 15 min after HFNC initiation (43.7% vs. 9%, $p = 0.04$) [41]. Lower oxygenation indices within the first hour of HFNC treatment were also found in those patients requiring intubation [41]. Schibler et al. [42] demonstrated in bronchiolitic infants a significant reduction in both heart rate and respiratory rate following commencement of HFNC. After 90 min on HFNC, the mean heart rate and respiratory rate each decreased by more than 20% of the baseline on these infants. Similarly, reduction in respiratory rate has been confirmed as an important predictor of HFNC success in other studies of infants and children [49–51]. This cumulative evidence suggests that if HFNC treatment is to succeed, this may be apparent very early in the course of HFNC therapy.

An important study from Roca and colleagues [46] combined the aforementioned data pertaining to adult patients into a tool, the ROX index, to assist in predicting the need for mechanical ventilation in patients with acute hypoxaemic respiratory failure receiving HFNC. The ROX index is a pneumonic for 'Respiratory rate-OXygenation', which is the ratio of SpO_2/FIO_2 to respiratory rate. The index was found not to have good predictive capacity at 2 or 6 h after HFNC initiation. However, after 12 h of HFNC, a ROX index of 4.88 or higher was associated with a lower risk for mechanical ventilation even after adjusting for potential confounding. At 12 h, the tool had a sensitivity of 70%, a specificity of 72%, a positive predictive value of 89%, and a negative predictive value of 42%. In the cohort of 157 patients on which the tool was tested, only 8.9% ($n = 14$) required intubation within 12 h of HFNC commencement. The ROX index appears to be an effective tool at predicting mechanical ventilation in adult patients with pneumonia leading to hypoxaemic acute respiratory failure. However, given the early indicators of failure mentioned above and the low rate of early non-responders in the study, it would be of great interest to further validate the predictive value of this index.

2.4.6 Patient Compliance with HFNC Therapy

On the whole, HFNC therapy is an extremely well-tolerated treatment modality and there are a number of factors which are likely to contribute to the high compliance rate. Humidification improves tolerability of oxygen therapy [5, 19] and therefore patient compliance. Additionally, face masks, and particularly the sealed face masks used to deliver NIV, make it difficult to communicate, drink and eat whereas HFNC therapy does not restrict these activities. Furthermore, enhanced comfort of HFNC when compared to face mask [26, 52, 53] and NIV [52, 54] makes the wearer more likely to continue with therapy. Tolerability of HFNC therapy was compared with NIV [48] and high-flow face mask [55] and, in both comparisons, HFNC was rated by patients as significantly more tolerable than the alternative delivery device.

However, in a randomised crossover study in patients with chronic obstructive pulmonary disease receiving home oxygen, participants reported poorer tolerance of HFNC than their home-use low-flow nasal prongs [56].

Reports from the literature regarding patients unable to continue with HFNC therapy are few. In the large majority of trials, authors report that no patient discontinued treatment. However, Parke and colleagues [57] in a randomised controlled trial of 340 patients reported that 12% (n = 20) of patients in the HFNC intervention arm were not able to continue therapy, with 12 of these reporting excessive heat as the reason. Similarly, Kim et al. [43] reported that 9% (n = 3) of patients had HFNC discontinued due to intolerance; however the specific reason was not given.

Simple measures employed to ensure compliance with HFNC therapy include correctly sized cannulae which sit comfortably within the nares; adequate humidification, particularly on initiation of the therapy when there may be a tendency to apply the cannulae before the humidifier has come up to temperature; reducing the humidifier temperature slightly if able in patients who find the heated gas uncomfortable; and providing adequate education to the patient, specifically regarding what to expect during the treatment particularly the sensation of heat, humidity and flow on commencement which some patients describe as unpleasant or uncomfortable.

Limited evidence exists for patient tolerance specifically relating to infants and children; however studies performed in the field of premature infants have indicated that HFNC therapy is better tolerated than NIV by the patient [58]. Importantly, the application of HFNC therapy allows the parent/carer to interact with the child much more and be able to perform cares for their child. This is both advantageous for the parent and the child.

2.5   Nursing Care Considerations

2.5.1   Skin Care and Oral Hygiene during HFNC Therapy

HFNC have a lower rate of interface-related pressure injuries compared to the face masks used to deliver NIV [59] but the skin and mucosa beneath the HFNC interface require regular inspection to identify any pressure-related injuries early. Additionally, the tops of the ears should be regularly inspected for signs of pressure injury from the head strap used to secure the cannula. Regular eye and mouth cares should be performed to minimise mucosal irritation or eye injury.

2.5.2   Activities of Daily Living

With HFNC, patients can communicate, eat and drink without interruption to therapy. The risk of aspiration is small and there is no published evidence of this occurring with HFNC use but, at high flow rates, it is a possibility. If tolerated by the adult patient, the flow rate could be decreased whilst eating or drinking to minimise this happening. This practice is strongly encouraged in the less-than-12-month age group due to the higher risk of aspiration. Normal sleep patterns should be encouraged whilst on HFNC therapy and, compared to NIV, adult patients report an improved quality sleep [60]. Depending on the device used to deliver HFNC therapy, an external battery may allow mobilisation. If battery backup is not available, exercise within the confines of the inspiratory circuit length should be encouraged. In some delivery systems there is the ability to use a connector for transporting the patient on HFNC via standard oxygen. In children with mild-to-moderate severity of illness this is tolerated well for short intra-hospital transfers only. Once the destination has been reached, they must be returned to higher flows with the HFNC delivery system.

2.5.3 Documentation

Regular documented observations of the patient are important, particularly on commencement of therapy. HFNC settings (flow and FiO_2) should be regularly documented as well as checking of the circuit, interface and humidifier settings. At a minimum, physiological observations should include respiratory rate, oxygen saturation and heart rate. It may be useful to document patient-reported dyspnoea levels to track subjective response to HFNC therapy. The condition of the skin under the HFNC interface should also be documented to ensure that no pressure-related injuries develop.

2.6 Conclusion

HFNC are increasingly used in critical and acute care settings to deliver respiratory support to patients of all ages. They are easy to set up and use; are well tolerated by patients; and have few reported adverse events. More research is required investigating optimal settings for HFNC initiation, maintenance and weaning, with specific aetiologies of respiratory failure in mind.

References

1. Franklin D, Babl FE, Schlapbach LJ, Oakley E, Craig S, Neutze J, et al. A randomized trial of high-flow oxygen therapy in infants with bronchiolitis. N Engl J Med. 2018;378:1121–31.
2. Ward JJ. High-flow oxygen administration by nasal cannula for adult and perinatal patients. Respir Care. 2013;58:98–122.
3. Wilkinson DJ, Andersen CC, Smith K, Holberton J. Pharyngeal pressure with high-flow nasal cannulae in premature infants. J Perinatol. 2008;28:42–7.
4. Mikalsen IB, Davis P, Oymar K. High flow nasal cannula in children: a literature review. Scand J Trauma Resusc Emerg Med. 2016;24:93.
5. Chanques G, Constantin JM, Sauter M, Jung B, Sebbane M, Verzilli D, et al. Discomfort associated with underhumidified high-flow oxygen therapy in critically ill patients. Intensive Care Med. 2009;35:996–1003.

6. Dysart K, Miller TL, Wolfson MR, Shaffer TH. Research in high flow therapy: mechanisms of action. Respir Med. 2009;103:1400–5.
7. L'Her E, Deye N, Lellouche F, Taille S, Demoule A, Fraticelli A, et al. Physiologic effects of noninvasive ventilation during acute lung injury. Am J Respir Crit Care Med. 2005;172:1112–8.
8. Bazuaye EA, Stone TN, Corris PA, Gibson GJ. Variability of inspired oxygen concentration with nasal cannulas. Thorax. 1992;47:609–11.
9. Ritchie JE, Williams AB, Gerard C, Hockey H. Evaluation of a humidified nasal high-flow oxygen system, using oxygraphy, capnography and measurement of upper airway pressures. Anaesth Intensive Care. 2011;39:1103–10.
10. Hough JL, Pham TM, Schibler A. Physiologic effect of high-flow nasal cannula in infants with bronchiolitis. Pediatr Crit Care Med. 2014;15:e214–9.
11. Hammer J, Numa A, Newth CJ. Acute respiratory distress syndrome caused by respiratory syncytial virus. Pediatr Pulmonol. 1997;23:176–83.
12. Pham TM, O'Malley L, Mayfield S, Martin S, Schibler A. The effect of high flow nasal cannula therapy on the work of breathing in infants with bronchiolitis. Pediatr Pulmonol. 2015;50:713–20.
13. Corley A, Caruana LR, Barnett AG, Tronstad O, Fraser JF. Oxygen delivery through high-flow nasal cannulae increase end-expiratory lung volume and reduce respiratory rate in post-cardiac surgical patients. Br J Anaesth. 2011;107:998–1004.
14. Mauri T, Alban L, Turrini C, Cambiaghi B, Carlesso E, Taccone P, et al. Optimum support by high-flow nasal cannula in acute hypoxemic respiratory failure: effects of increasing flow rates. Intensive Care Med. 2017;43:1453–63.
15. Parke RL, Bloch A, McGuinness SP. Effect of very-high-flow nasal therapy on airway pressure and end-expiratory lung impedance in healthy volunteers. Respir Care. 2015;60:1397–403.
16. Fontanari P, Burnet H, Zattara-Hartmann MC, Jammes Y. Changes in airway resistance induced by nasal inhalation of cold dry, dry, or moist air in normal individuals. J Appl Physiol (1985). 1996;81:1739–43.
17. Fontanari P, Zattara-Hartmann MC, Burnet H, Jammes Y. Nasal eupnoeic inhalation of cold, dry air increases airway resistance in asthmatic patients. Eur Respir J. 1997;10:2250–4.
18. Saslow JG, Aghai ZH, Nakhla TA, Hart JJ, Lawrysh R, Stahl GE, et al. Work of breathing using high-flow nasal cannula in preterm infants. J Perinatol. 2006;26:476–80.
19. Cuquemelle E, Pham T, Papon JF, Louis B, Danin PE, Brochard L. Heated and humidified high-flow oxygen therapy reduces discomfort during hypoxemic respiratory failure. Respir Care. 2012;57:1571–7.
20. Salah B, Dinh Xuan AT, Fouilladieu JL, Lockhart A, Regnard J. Nasal mucociliary transport in healthy subjects is slower when breathing dry air. Eur Respir J. 1988;1:852–5.
21. Hasani A, Chapman TH, McCool D, Smith RE, Dilworth JP, Agnew JE. Domiciliary humidification improves lung mucociliary clearance in patients with bronchiectasis. Chron Respir Dis. 2008;5:81–6.
22. Chikata Y, Izawa M, Okuda N, Itagaki T, Nakataki E, Onodera M, et al. Humidification performance of two high-flow nasal cannula devices: a bench study. Respir Care. 2014;59:1186–90.
23. Klompas M, Branson R, Eichenwald EC, Greene LR, Howell MD, Lee G, et al. Strategies to prevent ventilator-associated pneumonia in acute care hospitals: 2014 update. Infect Control Hosp Epidemiol. 2014;35(Suppl 2):S133–54.
24. Chikata Y, Unai K, Izawa M, Okuda N, Oto J, Nishimura M. Inspiratory tube condensation during high-flow nasal cannula therapy: a bench study. Respir Care. 2016;61:300–5.
25. Nishimura M. High-flow nasal cannula oxygen therapy in adults: physiological benefits, indication, clinical benefits, and adverse effects. Respir Care. 2016;61:529–41.
26. Maggiore SM, Idone FA, Vaschetto R, Festa R, Cataldo A, Antonicelli F, et al. Nasal high-flow versus Venturi mask oxygen therapy after extubation. Effects on oxygenation, comfort, and clinical outcome. Am J Respir Crit Care Med. 2014;190:282–8.
27. Nagata K, Kikuchi T, Horie T, Shiraki A, Kitajima T, Kadowaki T, et al. Domiciliary high-flow nasal cannula oxygen therapy for patients with stable Hypercapnic chronic obstructive pulmonary disease. A multicenter randomized crossover trial. Ann Am Thorac Soc. 2018;15:432–9.

28. Yu Y, Qian X, Liu C, Zhu C. Effect of high-flow nasal cannula versus conventional oxygen therapy for patients with thoracoscopic lobectomy after extubation. Can Respir J. 2017;2017:7894631.
29. Inoue S, Tamaki Y, Sonobe S, Egawa J, Kawaguchi M. A pediatric case developing critical abdominal distension caused by a combination of humidified high-flow nasal cannula oxygen therapy and nasal airway. JA Clin Rep. 2018;4:4.
30. Hegde S, Prodhan P. Serious air leak syndrome complicating high-flow nasal cannula therapy: a report of 3 cases. Pediatrics. 2013;131:e939–44.
31. Kang BJ, Koh Y, Lim CM, Huh JW, Baek S, Han M, et al. Failure of high-flow nasal cannula therapy may delay intubation and increase mortality. Intensive Care Med. 2015;41:623–32.
32. Carrillo A, Gonzalez-Diaz G, Ferrer M, Martinez-Quintana ME, Lopez-Martinez A, Llamas N, et al. Non-invasive ventilation in community-acquired pneumonia and severe acute respiratory failure. Intensive Care Med. 2012;38:458–66.
33. Moretti M, Cilione C, Tampieri A, Fracchia C, Marchioni A, Nava S. Incidence and causes of non-invasive mechanical ventilation failure after initial success. Thorax. 2000;55:819–25.
34. Pirret AM, Takerei SF, Matheson CL, Kelly M, Strickland W, Harford J, et al. Nasal high flow oxygen therapy in the ward setting: a prospective observational study. Intensive Crit Care Nurs. 2017;42:127–34.
35. Plate JDJ, Leenen LPH, Platenkamp M, Meijer J, Hietbrink F. Introducing high-flow nasal cannula oxygen therapy at the intermediate care unit: expanding the range of supportive pulmonary care. Trauma Surg Acute Care Open. 2018;3:e000179.
36. Storgaard LH, Hockey H-U, Laursen BS, Weinreich UM. Long-term effects of oxygen-enriched high-flow nasal cannula treatment in COPD patients with chronic hypoxemic respiratory failure. Int J Chron Obstruct Pulmon Dis. 2018;13:1195–205.
37. Bressan S, Balzani M, Krauss B, Pettenazzo A, Zanconato S, Baraldi E. High-flow nasal cannula oxygen for bronchiolitis in a pediatric ward: a pilot study. Eur J Pediatr. 2013;172:1649–56.
38. Schibler A, Franklin D. Respiratory support for children in the emergency department. J Paediatr Child Health. 2016;52:192–6.
39. Spoletini G, Alotaibi M, Blasi F, Hill NS. Heated humidified high-flow nasal oxygen in adults: mechanisms of action and clinical implications. Chest. 2015;148:253–61.
40. Ischaki E, Pantazopoulos I, Zakynthinos S. Nasal high flow therapy: a novel treatment rather than a more expensive oxygen device. Eur Respir Rev. 2017;26:170028.
41. Sztrymf B, Messika J, Bertrand F, Hurel D, Leon R, Dreyfuss D, et al. Beneficial effects of humidified high flow nasal oxygen in critical care patients: a prospective pilot study. Intensive Care Med. 2011;37:1780–6.
42. Schibler A, Pham TM, Dunster KR, Foster K, Barlow A, Gibbons K, et al. Reduced intubation rates for infants after introduction of high-flow nasal prong oxygen delivery. Intensive Care Med. 2011;37:847–52.
43. Kim ES, Lee H, Kim SJ, Park J, Lee YJ, Park JS, et al. Effectiveness of high-flow nasal cannula oxygen therapy for acute respiratory failure with hypercapnia. J Thorac Dis. 2018;10:882–8.
44. Koga Y, Kaneda K, Mizuguchi I, Nakahara T, Miyauchi T, Fujita M, et al. Extent of pleural effusion on chest radiograph is associated with failure of high-flow nasal cannula oxygen therapy. J Crit Care. 2016;32:165–9.
45. Messika J, Ben Ahmed K, Gaudry S, Miguel-Montanes R, Rafat C, Sztrymf B, et al. Use of high-flow nasal cannula oxygen therapy in subjects with ARDS: a 1-year observational study. Respir Care. 2015;60:162–9.
46. Roca O, Messika J, Caralt B, Garcia-de-Acilu M, Sztrymf B, Ricard JD, et al. Predicting success of high-flow nasal cannula in pneumonia patients with hypoxemic respiratory failure: the utility of the ROX index. J Crit Care. 2016;35:200–5.
47. Rello J, Perez M, Roca O, Poulakou G, Souto J, Laborda C, et al. High-flow nasal therapy in adults with severe acute respiratory infection: a cohort study in patients with 2009 influenza a/H1N1v. J Crit Care. 2012;27:434–9.

48. Frat JP, Brugiere B, Ragot S, Chatellier D, Veinstein A, Goudet V, et al. Sequential application of oxygen therapy via high-flow nasal cannula and noninvasive ventilation in acute respiratory failure: an observational pilot study. Respir Care. 2015;60:170–8.
49. Abboud PA, Roth PJ, Skiles CL, Stolfi A, Rowin ME. Predictors of failure in infants with viral bronchiolitis treated with high-flow, high-humidity nasal cannula therapy*. Pediatr Crit Care Med. 2012;13:e343–9.
50. Kelly GS, Simon HK, Sturm JJ. High-flow nasal cannula use in children with respiratory distress in the emergency department: predicting the need for subsequent intubation. Pediatr Emerg Care. 2013;29:888–92.
51. Mayfield S, Bogossian F, O'Malley L, Schibler A. High-flow nasal cannula oxygen therapy for infants with bronchiolitis: pilot study. J Paediatr Child Health. 2014;50:373–8.
52. Frat JP, Thille AW, Mercat A, Girault C, Ragot S, Perbet S, et al. High-flow oxygen through nasal cannula in acute hypoxemic respiratory failure. N Engl J Med. 2015;372:2185–96.
53. Roca O, Riera J, Torres F, Masclans JR. High-flow oxygen therapy in acute respiratory failure. Respir Care. 2010;55:408–13.
54. Schwabbauer N, Berg B, Blumenstock G, Haap M, Hetzel J, Riessen R. Nasal high–flow oxygen therapy in patients with hypoxic respiratory failure: effect on functional and subjective respiratory parameters compared to conventional oxygen therapy and non-invasive ventilation (NIV). BMC Anesthesiol. 2014;14:66.
55. Tiruvoipati R, Lewis D, Haji K, Botha J. High-flow nasal oxygen vs high-flow face mask: a randomized crossover trial in extubated patients. J Crit Care. 2010;25:463–8.
56. Fraser JF, Spooner AJ, Dunster KR, Anstey CM, Corley A. Nasal high flow oxygen therapy in patients with COPD reduces respiratory rate and tissue carbon dioxide while increasing tidal and end-expiratory lung volumes: a randomised crossover trial. Thorax. 2016;71:759–61.
57. Parke R, McGuinness S, Dixon R, Jull A. Open-label, phase II study of routine high-flow nasal oxygen therapy in cardiac surgical patients. Br J Anaesth. 2013;111:925–31.
58. Manley BJ, Owen LS, Doyle LW, Andersen CC, Cartwright DW, Pritchard MA, et al. High-flow nasal cannulae in very preterm infants after extubation. N Engl J Med. 2013;369:1425–33.
59. Stephan F, Barrucand B, Petit P, Rezaiguia-Delclaux S, Medard A, Delannoy B, et al. High-flow nasal oxygen vs noninvasive positive airway pressure in hypoxemic patients after cardiothoracic surgery: a randomized clinical trial. JAMA. 2015;313:2331–9.
60. Hui D, Morgado M, Chisholm G, Withers L, Nguyen Q, Finch C, et al. High-flow oxygen and bilevel positive airway pressure for persistent dyspnea in patients with advanced cancer: a phase II randomized trial. J Pain Symptom Manag. 2013;46:463–73.

Physiological Effects of High Flow in Adults

3

Francesca Dalla Corte, Irene Ottaviani, Giacomo Montanari, Yu Mei Wang, and Tommaso Mauri

3.1 Introduction

High-flow nasal cannula (HFNC) is a noninvasive respiratory support designed to deliver 30–60 L/min of a heated, humidified mixture of air and oxygen through specifically designed nasal prongs. Previous studies showed that HFNC is associated with multiple physiological effects, ranging from improved lung volumes to decreased work of breathing to optimal humidification of airways. In this chapter, we summarize relevant effects in adult patients (Fig. 3.1).

3.2 Physiological Effects in Healthy Subjects

In healthy volunteers [1], the set flow rate of HFNC has a positive linear correlation with the low level of positive pressure generated in the upper airways, whether the mouth is open or closed. HFNC delivered at 0, 10, 20, 40, and 60 L/min with the mouth closed generates mean airway pressure of 0.8, 1.7, 2.9, 5.5, and 7.7 cmH$_2$O, respectively. Similar linear increase of pressure effect was reported in the research by Ritchie et al. [2] and Corley et al. in hypoxemic patients, too [3].

F. Dalla Corte · I. Ottaviani · G. Montanari
Morphology, Surgery and Experimental Medicine, Anesthesia and Intensive Care Unit, University of Ferrara, Ferrara, Italy

Y. M. Wang
Department of Critical Care Medicine, Beijing Tiantan Hospital, Capital Medical University, Beijing, China

T. Mauri (✉)
Department of Pathophysiology and Transplantation, University of Milan, Milan, Italy

Department of Anesthesia, Critical Care and Emergency, Foundation IRCCS Ca' Granda Maggiore PoliclinicoHospital, Milan, Italy
e-mail: tommaso.mauri@unimi.it

© Springer Nature Switzerland AG 2021   55
A. Carlucci, S. M. Maggiore (eds.), *High Flow Nasal Cannula*,
https://doi.org/10.1007/978-3-030-42454-1_3

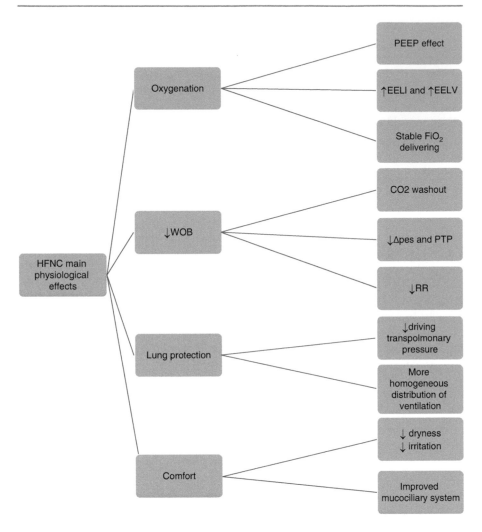

Fig. 3.1 Main physiological effects of HFNC therapy

A positive linear correlation exists between the amount of flow delivered and the resulting airway pressure generated with conventional flows of 30–50 L/min. Parke et al. [4] performed a study on healthy volunteers to test if the correlation remains linear at flows exceeding 50 L/min. Fifteen healthy volunteers were recruited and positive linear relationship was described between gas flow rate up to 100 L/min and mean airway pressure. On average, for every 10 L/min increase in gas flow, the generated mean airway pressure increased by 1.16 cmH$_2$O. At the maximum flow of 100 L/min, the mean airway pressure was 11.9 ± 2.7 cmH$_2$O. As the gas flow was increased, there was an accompanying positive increase in the cumulative change in end-expiratory lung volume measured by electrical impedance tomography. Interestingly, the decrease in respiratory rate by HFNC plateaued at a flow of 50 L/min.

Recently, Mauri et al. [5] suggested a novel noninvasive support, the combination of HFNC+HELMET, in a small sample of healthy volunteers. The novel HFNC+HELMET system, delivering nasal high flow within a sealed helmet connected to a PEEP valve, provided clinically relevant, measurable, and stable positive airway pressure in healthy volunteers. Moreover, the HFNC+HELMET system granted effective CO_2 washout from the upper airways, with negligible CO_2 rebreathing. The combination of HFNC+HELMET might be a new and useful respiratory support in hypoxemic patients to grant positive airway pressure higher than HFNC coupled with effective CO_2 washout. Another study showed that the increase in lung volume by HFNC is also related to changes in body position. The Spanish group of Riera et al. [6] used electrical impedance tomography (EIT) to measure an increase in lung volume by HFNC among healthy subjects in the supine position and in the prone position. These findings were in agreement with Mauri et al. [7, 8] who showed that the use of HFNC in the semi-seated position in subjects with acute hypoxemic respiratory failure improved lung volume (see below). In 2018, Plotnikow et al. [9] assessed lung volume change induced by HFNC at different flow rates in healthy subjects in the supine and semi-seated position. Global lung volume was significantly different among all the conditions and increased from 0 in supine position to 1.05 (0.72–1.34) units in the semi-seated position and further increased to 1.12 (0.8–2.01) units and 1.44 (1.05–2.16) units, increasing the flow from 30 to 50 L/min in the semi-seated position. Regionally, the ratio of lung volume in dependent and nondependent regions increased from 0.6 to 0.78 with HFNC at 50 L/min, indicating more homogeneous inflation. Perez-Teràn and colleagues performed a study on healthy subjects comparing the effects of positive-pressure NIV with HFNC using electrical impedance tomography: no differences were found on RR and lung volume, but NIV significantly increased nondependent silent spaces (indicating overdistension), while aeration changes during HFNC were more homogeneous [10].

The other relevant effect in healthy subjects is the decrease in respiratory rate by HFNC. Riera et al. [6] described a significant decrease in the breathing frequency when HFNC was implemented, in both supine and prone positions. In the supine position there was a mean decrease of 2.73 breaths/min (95% CI 0.4-5.08, $p = 0.02$) from ambient air to HFNC. In the prone position, the mean decrease was 7.89 breaths/min (95% CI 4.38–11.4, $p = 0.001$). Plotnikow et al. [9] also disclosed a decline in respiratory rate among healthy subjects, but the decline was more pronounced (a decrease of 4.4 and 6.3 breaths/min for flow of 30 and 50 L/min, respectively) compared with patients studied by Mauri et al. (2 breaths/min), Corley et al. (3.4 breaths/min), or Riera et al. (2.7 breaths/min) [3, 5, 6]. Comparing HFNC to no support, Okuda et al. [11] found that respiratory rate decreased (off vs. 30 vs. 50 L/min: 15.1 ± 2.14 bpm vs. 11.6 ± 3.08 bpm vs. 11.1 ± 2.29 bpm), too. However, the decrease was negligible between 30 and 50 L/min. The rapid shallow breathing index (RSBI, ratio of the respiratory frequency to tidal volume) showed a significant tendency to decrease with the HFNC, compared with no support. Bräunlich et al. [12] and Mündel et al. [13] also described a similar pattern with decreased respiratory rate. The main mechanism may be the reduction of the anatomic dead space generated by the CO_2 washout effect.

As far as inspiratory tidal volume is concerned, the results seem mixed. Okuda et al. [11] demonstrated that tidal volume markedly increased at increasing flow rates (no support vs. 30 L/min vs. 50 L/min: 685.6 ± 236.5 mL vs. 929.8 ± 434.7 mL vs. 968.8 ± 451.1 mL). Bräunlich et al. [12] and Mündel et al. [13] used an elastic sensor belt for polysomnography to measure tidal volume in healthy volunteers. Interestingly, the two papers provided different results. In the study by Mündel et al., HFNC led to a marked increase in tidal volume associated with a reduction in respiratory rate during wakefulness. There was no change in overall minute ventilation between HFNC and baseline. In contrast, during sleep, the authors described a fall in minute ventilation due to a decrease in tidal volume without change in RR. The reduction in tidal volume, however, was associated with stable oxyhemoglobin level (SaO_2). In Bräunlich's trial, tidal volume was decreased in healthy volunteers during HFNC, while it increased in patients with chronic obstructive pulmonary disease; in both groups respiratory rate and minute ventilation decreased. Age, sex, clinical condition, and the method to measure tidal volume may account for these differences.

Finally, HFNC, delivering heated and humidified air/oxygen, provides more comfort to the patients, both in healthy subjects and in hypoxemic patients. Moreover, HFNC guarantees effective clearance of the secretion, preserving the function of the mucociliary system, and decreases the incidence of eye irritation and dryness of the upper airway's mucosa [8, 14–16].

3.3 Physiological Effects in Hypoxemic Patients

HFNC is indicated to support patients with acute hypoxemic respiratory failure (AHRF) since the low level of positive airway pressure may have several benefits including alveolar recruitment, improved ventilation/perfusion matching, reduced airway resistance, and reduced work of breathing. Moreover, HFNC may improve oxygenation by decreasing oxygen dilution due to the high inspiratory flow, decreasing dead space [17], and providing high levels of humidification.

3.3.1 Positive Airway Pressure and Increase in End-Expiratory Lung Volume

As showed in healthy volunteers and in infants, Parke et al. [18] studied a cohort of postoperative cardiac surgery adult patients undergoing HFNC and described a statistically significant effect on nasopharyngeal pressure compared to standard face mask. Mean positive values of nasopharyngeal pressure varied between $1.2 ± 0.76$ cmH$_2$O (mouth open) and $2.7 ± 1.04$ cmH$_2$O (mouth closed) and both were higher than values obtained with face mask. Corley et al. [3] described significant positive correlation ($r = 0.7$, $p = 0.001$) between nasopharyngeal pressure and end-expiratory lung volume measured by electrical impedance tomography.

HFNC at 35 L/min increased airway pressure by a mean value of 3.0 cmH$_2$O compared to low-flow oxygen, with a corresponding mean increase in lung volume of 25.6%. Mauri et al. [7] showed a global increase in lung volume with HFNC set at 40 L/min compared to face mask oxygenation in a cohort of AHRF patients. This increase in lung volume was associated with an improvement of global inhomogeneity ventilation index indicating more homogeneous distribution of ventilation throughout the lungs. Moreover, they found a reduction in patients' peak expiratory flow (PEF) in the dependent lung regions ($-34 \pm 18\%$, $p < 0.001$), as an indirect sign of improvement of lung compliance in that region. In a subsequent study Mauri et al. [19] described that lung volume increased linearly with the set flow rate (from low-flow oxygen to 30, 45, and 60 L/min with HFNC). The increase in lung volume was mainly due to linear improvement of the regional end-expiratory volume in the dependent regions. Since this was associated with a linear increase in dynamic lung compliance and peripheral arterial oxygenation, the authors hypothesized that positive pressure effect by HFNC might have induced regional recruitment.

3.3.2 Reduction in Work of Breathing

Respiratory muscle activity in AHRF increases due to the high respiratory drive. Unassisted spontaneous breathing might be "a double-edged sword" [20], with the generation of higher trans-pulmonary pressure [21] and muscle fatigue. Hence, noninvasive support should preserve the lung from superimposed injuries while unloading inspiratory muscles. Sztrymf et al. [22] were the first to evaluate the effects of HFNC on the work of breathing in a cohort of patients failing conventional oxygen therapy. Fifteen minutes after the beginning of HFNC they described an improvement of respiratory rate and a significant reduction in heart rate, dyspnea score, supraclavicular retraction, and thoracoabdominal asynchrony, coupled with a significant improvement in pulse oximetry. No signs of discomfort were present. These results were later confirmed by Itakagi et al. [23]: HFNC therapy was associated with a decrease in respiratory rate and an improvement in thoracoabdominal synchrony measured by respiratory inductive plethysmography compared to facial mask standard oxygen. Mauri et al. [7] then described how during HFNC at 40 L/min esophageal pressure swings (ΔPes) were significantly lower (HFNC 8.0 $\pm$ 3.4 vs. LFOT 9.9 $\pm$ 4.2 cmH$_2$O, $p < 0.01$) compared to low-flow oxygen, indicating that patients had less inspiratory effort. They also pointed out that the tidal volume/ΔPes ratio (i.e., an estimate of the dynamic lung compliance) was significantly higher during HFNC ($p < 0.05$), possibly indicating external "ventilation support" by the mandatory flow of HFNC during inspiration, improved lung mechanics, or both. Pressure time product (PTP) was also significantly lower with HFNC, suggesting lighter metabolic work of breathing. The same group later showed [19] how increasing HFNC flow rates progressively decreased respiratory rate ($p < 0.01$) in comparison to standard facial mask. Similarly, the inspiratory effort as measured by ΔPes and PTP decreased significantly by application of HFNC at increasing flows

($p < 0.001$ for both). However, most of the benefit was measured when switching from facial mask to HFNC, while further increase in flow rate did not lead to additional improvement. Twelve patients with AHRF were studied by Vargas et al. [24] comparing the effect on WOB of conventional O_2 therapy vs. HFNC and CPAP (5 cmH_2O): PTP was lower during HFNC and CPAP compared to conventional O_2 and there was a decrease in airway resistance and an improvement in oxygenation. Despite these positive physiological results, we must point out that in all these studies variability between patients was very high and the optimum personalized flow should be titrated at the bedside (possibly starting from the highest downwards). Maggiore et al. compared HFNC with Venturi mask in 105 hypoxic patients after extubation. Results showed an improvement in oxygenation in the treatment group (50 L/min) at 24, 36, and 48 h, probably due to lung recruitment of atelectatic zones and oxygen reservoir created by the flow in the upper airways. Furthermore, CO_2 washout decreased the respiratory drive and dyspnea [25].

The positive clinical results in hypoxemic patients reported by Frat et al. [26], and in post-extubation period by Hernandez et al. [25, 27], might be due to the improved lung protection by positive airway pressure effect coupled with muscle unloading by the CO_2 washout.

Interestingly, studies on tracheostomized patients, despite noticing an improvement in oxygenation, probably due to more stable alveolar FiO_2, showed no significant improvement in inspiratory effort during high-flow therapy through the tracheostomy cannula (T-HF) [28, 29]. Indeed, one of the major effects of HFNC is the washout effect and the positive pressure generated through the airway, mechanisms that could be reduced or absent bypassing the larynx and the upper airways as with T-HF.

3.4   Physiological Effects in Chronic Patients

Chronic obstructive pulmonary disease (COPD) is the fourth leading cause of chronic morbidity [30, 31]. To date, noninvasive ventilation (NIV) and long-term oxygen therapy (LTOT) are the preferred options for hypoxemic and hypercapnic patients with COPD. The current recommendations for LTOT prescription in COPD patients are based on the results of two randomized trials published almost 30 years ago: the Medical Research Council (MRC) study [32] and the Nocturnal Oxygen Therapy Trial (NOTT) [33]. The results of both studies indicated that continuous LTOT was better than nocturnal LTOT and that LTOT conferred a significant survival benefit in COPD patients with resting hypoxemia [34]. The role of long-term NIV in chronic hypercapnic respiratory failure due to COPD is more controversial. Recently, the work of Raveling et al. found no survival benefit in a cohort of patients affected by hypercapnic COPD treated with chronic NIV [35]. In recent years, high-flow nasal cannula (HFNC) therapy gained attention as an alternative respiratory support in COPD because of the theoretical benefits associated to its physiological effects. Here we summarize the most relevant.

3.4.1   Improved Mucociliary Clearance, Positive Airway Pressure, and Increase in End-Expiratory Lung Volume

The beneficial effects on mucociliary clearance of the heated and humidified HFNC gas flow were underlined by Chidekel et al. in epithelial respiratory cell culture. The authors compared inflammatory cytokine production and change in cell morphology between three groups of cells exposed to different levels of relative humidity (RH) (20% RH, the "dry group," 69% RH, 90% RH, the HFNC group) at a temperature of 37°. They found an increase in cytokine production and high percentage of morphological abnormalities of epithelial cells (puffed nuclei, intracellular and nuclear vacuoles, diffuse cytoplasm, and cellular detritus) in the dry group, compared to the other [36]. In vivo, these results were initially tested in patients with bronchiectasis. In particular, Hasani et al. showed how in this population treatment for 3 h/day for 7 consecutive days at a flow of 20–25 L/min at 37° increased lung clearance, measured by the amount of peripheral deposition of the radio-pulmonary aerosols (99 m Tc) compared with baseline [37].

Another physiological hallmark of COPD patients is exercise intolerance, mainly due to high dead space of upper airways causing an increase in minute ventilation. A study showed that HFNC could mitigate this effect by washing out the CO_2 [38].

Although HFNC is an open system, it could provide a moderate level of positive airway pressure, correlated with the set flow rate and with the ratio between nasal prong size and nostrils. This effect has been confirmed in healthy volunteers [39], stable COPD and idiopathic pulmonary fibrosis [12], and postcardiac surgery patients [3]. As mentioned before, the amount of positive pressure generated by HFNC has been studied in healthy volunteers and in patients [18] through direct measure in the nasopharyngeal space and increased end-expiratory lung volume [6–9]. We can argue that the modest quote of positive airway pressure generated by HFNC is transmitted to the lower respiratory tract with the effect of increasing the functional residual capacity.

3.4.2   Reduction in Work of Breathing

In COPD patients, the intrinsic PEEP generated by collapse of small airways during expiration increases the work of breathing (WOB): thus, the positive airway pressure generated by HFNC could counterbalance the intrinsic PEEP and reduce the respiratory workload. A study [40] in which standard oxygen therapy was compared to HFNC in stable hypercapnic COPD patients found a decrease in respiratory muscle effort when comparing HFNC with standard oxygen therapy; in addition, trans-diaphragmatic pressure swing (Pdi) and pressure time product of the diaphragm (PTPdi) were reduced as well as respiratory rate and $PaCO_2$ levels. Di Mussi et al. [41] performed a study on COPD patients extubated after mechanical ventilation initiated for hypercapnic respiratory failure. They enrolled 14 patients to study the neuro-ventilatory drive, assessed by electrical activity of the diaphragm (EAdi) and work of breathing, assessed by the PTP, during HFNC therapy and standard O_2

therapy. The patients underwent three phases: one phase (1 h) of HFNC therapy with flow increasing from 20 L/min to the highest tolerated value (max 60 L/min), one phase (1 h) of standard O_2 therapy with facial mask (10 L/min), and last phase (1 h) of HFNC. Both EAdi and PTP increased significantly during conventional O_2 phase compared with HFNC phases, suggesting decreased respiratory drive and work of breathing that could lead to decreased risk of weaning failure. Braunlich et al. [42] recruited 67 hospitalized patients with COPD in order to study the effect of HFNC, nBiPAP, nCPAP, and standard oxygen therapy. During HFNC, increased flow was related to a proportional increase in airway pressure (20 L/min: 0.92 ± 0.49 mbar; 30 L/min: 1.44 ± 0.78 mbar; 40 L/min: 2.14 ± 0.98 mbar; 50 L/min: 3.01 ± 1.03 mbar) and in tidal volume, and a decrease in respiratory and rapid shallow breathing. Moreover, $PaCO_2$ decreased with increasing flow from 20 L/min (91 ± 6.7 mmHg) to 30 L/min (87 ± 6.2 mmHg, $p < 0.03$). The same group recruited 36 COPD patients to receive in random order HFNC therapy with different flows and leakage conditions; they described that, by increasing flow, airway pressure increased but $PaCO_2$ was not linearly related to the airway pressure. At the opposite, an increase in the % of leak yielding a decrease in mean airway pressure resulted in the lowest $PaCO_2$ level [43]. This study might confirm the previous results on the relationship between leakage and CO_2 washout effect in animal model [44].

However, randomized control trials on the use of HFNC in COPD are still lacking and, despite sound physiological rationale, use in this population should be careful and in a monitored environment.

3.5 Conclusions

In conclusion, HFNC is increasingly used in the management of acute respiratory failure due to the multiple physiological benefits, the ease of use, and the elevated patients' compliance to treatment.

Acknowledgements
Conflicts of Interest: TM reports personal fees from Fisher & Paykel, Drager, Mindray. The other authors do not have any conflict to disclose.

References

1. Groves N, Tobin A. High flow nasal oxygen generates positive airway pressure in adult volunteers. Aust Crit Care. 2007;20(4):126–31.
2. Ritchie JE, Williams AB, Gerard C. Evaluation of a high flow nasal oxygenation system: gas analysis and pharyngeal pressures. Intensive Care Med. 2006;32:S219.
3. Corley A, Caruana LR, Barnett AG, Tronstad O, Fraser JF. Oxygen delivery through high-flow nasal cannulae increase end-expiratory lung volume and reduce respiratory rate in post-cardiac surgical patients. Br J Anaesth. 2011;107(6):998–1004.
4. Parke RL, Bloch A, McGuinness SP. Effect of very-high-flow nasal therapy on airway pressure and end-expiratory lung impedance in healthy volunteers. Respir Care. 2015;60:1397.

5. Mauri T, Spinelli E, Mariani M, Guzzardella A, Del Prete C, Carlesso E, Tortolani D, Tagliabue P, Pesenti A, Grasselli G. Nasal high flow delivered within the helmet: a new non-invasive respiratory support. AJRCCM. 2018;199:1.

6. Riera J, Perez P, Cortes J, Roca O, Masclans JR, Rello J. Effect of high-flow nasal cannula and body position on end-expiratory lung volume: a cohort study using electrical impedance tomography. Respir Care. 2013;58(4):589–96.

7. Mauri T, Turrini C, Eronia N, Grasselli G, Volta CA, Bellani G, et al. Physiologic effects of high-flow nasal cannula in acute hypoxemic respiratory failure. Am J Respir Crit Care Med. 2017;195(9):1207–15.

8. Mauri T, Galazzi A, Binda F, Masciopinto L, Corcione N, Carlesso E, et al. Impact of flow and temperature on patient comfort during respiratory support by high-flow nasal cannula. Crit care (London, England). *2018*;22(*1*):*120.*

9. Plotnikow GA, Thille AW, Vasquez DN, Pratto RA, Quiroga CM, Andrich ME, et al. Effects of high-flow nasal cannula on end-expiratory lung impedance in semi-seated healthy subjects. Respir Care. 2018;63(8):1016–23.

10. Pérez-Terán P, Marin-Corral J, Dot I, et al. Aeration changes induced by high flow nasal cannula are more homogeneous than those generated by non-invasive ventilation in healthy subjects. J Crit Care. 2019;53:186–92.

11. Okuda M, Tanaka N, Naito K, Kumada T, Fukuda K, Kato Y, et al. Evaluation by various methods of the physiological mechanism of a high-flow nasal cannula (HFNC) in healthy volunteers. BMJ Open Respir Res. 2017;4(1):e000200.

12. Braunlich J, Beyer D, Mai D, Hammerschmidt S, Seyfarth HJ, Wirtz H. Effects of nasal high flow on ventilation in volunteers, COPD and idiopathic pulmonary fibrosis patients. Respiration. 2013;85(4):319–25.

13. Mundel T, Feng S, Tatkov S, Schneider H. Mechanisms of nasal high flow on ventilation during wakefulness and sleep. J Appl Physiol (1985). *2013*;114(8):1058–65.

14. Chanques G, Contantin JM, Sauter M, et al. Discomfort associated with underhumidified high-flow oxygen therapy in critically ill patients. Intensive Care Med. 2009;35(6):996–1003.

15. Andres D, Thurston N, Brant R, et al. Randomized double-blind trial of the effects of humidified compared with non-humidified low flow oxygen therapy on the symptoms of patients. Can Respir J. 1997;4:76–80.

16. Salah B, Dinh Xuan AT, Fouilladieu JL, et al. Nasal mucociliary transport in healthy subjects is slower when breathing dry air. Eur Respir J. 1988;1(9):852–5.

17. L'Her E, Deye N, Lellouche F, Taille S, Demoule A, Fraticelli A, Mancebo J, Brochard L. Physiologic effects of noninvasive ventilation during acute lung injury. Am J Respir Crit Care Med. 2005;172(9):1112–8.

18. Parke R, McGuinness S, Eccleston M. Nasal high-flow therapy delivers low level positive airway pressure. Br J Anaesth. 2009;103:886–90.

19. Mauri T, Alban L, Turrini C, Cambiaghi B, Carlesso E, Taccone P, Bottino N, Lissoni A, Spadaro S, Volta CA, Gattinoni L, Pesenti A, Grasselli G. Optimum support by high-flow nasal cannula in acute hypoxemic respiratory failure: effects of increasing flow rates. Intensive Care Med. 2017;43(10):1453–63.

20. Brochard L. Ventilation-induced lung injury exists in spontaneously breathing patients with acute respiratory failure: yes. Intensive Care Med. 2017;43:250–2.

21. Yoshida T, Uchiyama A, Matsuura N, et al. Spontaneous breathing during lung-protective ventilation in an experimental acute lung injury model: high transpulmonary pressure associated with strong spontaneous breathing effort may worsen lung injury. Crit Care Med. 2012;40:1578–85.

22. Sztrymf B, Messika J, Bertrand F, Hurel D, Leon R, Dreyfuss D, Ricard JD. Beneficial effects of humidified high flow nasal oxygen in critical care patients: a prospective pilot study. Intensive Care Med. 2011;37(11):1780–6.

23. Itagaki T, Okuda N, Tsunano Y, Kohata H, Nakataki E, Onodera M, Imanaka H, Nishimura M. Effect of high-flow nasal cannula on thoraco-abdominal synchrony in adult critically ill patients. Respir Care. 2014;59(1):70–4.

24. Vargas F, Saint-Leger M, Boyer A, Bui N, Hilbert G. Physiologic effects of high-flow nasal cannula oxygen in critical care subjects. Respir Care. 2015;60:1369.
25. Maggiore SM, Idone F, Vaschetto R, et al. Nasal high-flow vs venturi mask oxygen therapy after extubation: effects on oxygenation, comfort and clinical outcome. Am J Respir Crit Care Med. 2014:190. https://doi.org/10.1164/rccm.201402-0364OC.
26. Frat J-P, Thille A, Mercat A, Girault C, Ragot S, Perbet, et al. High-flow oxygen through nasal cannula in acute hypoxemic respiratory failure. New Engl J Med. 2015:372. https://doi.org/10.1056/NEJMoa1503326.
27. Hernández G, Vaquero C, Colinas L, et al. Effect of Postextubation high-flow nasal cannula vs noninvasive ventilation on reintubation and Postextubation respiratory failure in high-risk patients: a randomized clinical trial. JAMA. 2016;316(15):1565–74.
28. Hernández G, Vaquero C, González P, et al. Effect of postextubation high-flow nasal cannula vs conventional oxygen therapy on reintubation in low-risk patients: a randomized clinical trial. JAMA. 2016;315(13):1354–61.
29. Stripoli T, Spadaro S, Di Mussi R, et al. High-flow oxygen therapy in tracheostomized patients at high risk of weaning failure. Ann Intensive Care. 2019;9(1):4.
30. Corley A, Edwards M, Spooner AJ, Dunster KR, Anstey C, Fraser JF. High-flow oxygen via tracheostomy improves oxygenation in patients weaning from mechanical ventilation: a randomised crossover study. Intensive Care Med. 2017;43(3):465–7.
31. Jemal A, Ward E, Hao Y, Thun M. *Trends in the leading causes of death in the United States, 1970–2002*. JAMA. *2005;294:1255–9.*
32. Fang X, Wang X, Bai C. COPD in China: the burden and importance of proper management. Chest. 2011;139:920–9.
33. Report of the Medical Research Council Working Party Long term domiciliary oxygen therapy in chronic hypoxic cor pulmonale complicating chronic bronchitis and emphysema. Lancet. 1981;1(8222):681–6.
34. Nocturnal Oxygen Therapy Trial Group. Continuous or nocturnal oxygen therapy in hypoxemic chronic obstructive lung disease: a clinical trial. Ann Intern Med. 1980;93(3):391–8.
35. Stoller JK, Panos RJ, Krachman S, Doherty DE, Make B. Long-term oxygen treatment trial research group. Oxygen therapy for patients with COPD: current evidence and the long-term oxygen treatment trial. Chest. 2010;138(1):179–87.
36. Raveling T, Bladder G, Vonk JM, Nieuwenhuis JA, Verdonk-Struik FM, Wijkstra PJ, Duiverman ML. Improvement in hypercapnia does not predict survival in COPD patients on chronic noninvasive ventilation. Int J Chron Obstruct Pulmon Dis. 2018;13:3625–34.
37. Chidekel A, Zhu Y, Wang J, Mosko JJ, Rodriguez E, Shaffer TH. The effects of gas humidification with high-flow nasal cannula on cultured human airway epithelial cells. Pulm Med. 2012;2012:380686.
38. Hasani A, Chapman TH, McCool D, Smith RE, Dilworth JP, Agnew JE. Domiciliary humidification improves lung mucociliary clearance in patients with bronchiectasis. Chron Respir Dis. 2008;5:81–6.
39. Parke RL, Eccleston ML, McGuinness SP. The effects of flow on air- way pressure during nasal high-flow oxygen therapy. Respir Care. 2011;56:1151–5.
40. Sim MA, Dean P, Kinsella J, Black R, Carter R, Hughes M. Performance of oxygen delivery devices when the breathing pattern of respiratory failure is simulated. Anaesthesia. 2008;63:938–40.
41. Pisani L, Fasano L, Corcione N, Comellini V, Musti MA, Brandao M, et al. Change in pulmonary mechanics and the effect on breathing pat- tern of high flow oxygen therapy in stable hypercapnic COPD. Thorax. 2017;72:373–5.

42. Di Mussi R, Spadaro S, Stripoli T, Volta CA, Trerotoli P, Pierucci P, Staffieri F, Bruno F, Camporota L, Grasso S. High-flow nasal cannula oxygen therapy decreases postextubation neuroventilatory drive and work of breathing in patients with chronic obstructive pulmonary disease. Crit Care. 2018;22(*1*):*180*. https://doi.org/10.1186/s13054-018-2107-9. PMID: 30071876; PMCID: PMC6091018
43. Bräunlich J, Köhler M, Wirtz H. Nasal high flow improves ventilation in patients with COPD. Int J Chron Obstruct Pulmon Dis. 2016;11:1077–85.
44. Braunlich J, Mauersberger F, Wirtz H. Effectiveness of nasal high flow in hypercapnic COPD patients is flow and leakage dependent. BMC Pulm Med. 2018;18:14.

Clinical Applications of High-Flow Nasal Cannula in Acute Hypoxemic Respiratory Failure

4

Jean-Pierre Frat, Damien Marie, Jonathan Messika, and Jean-Damien Ricard

4.1 Introduction

To date, there is no well-established definition of acute respiratory failure. The criteria most widely used in clinical studies are a respiratory rate between 20 and 25 breaths/min, clinical signs of respiratory failure, and hypoxemia commonly defined with a PaO_2/FiO_2 ratio below 200 or 300 mm Hg. Acute hypoxemic or de novo respiratory failure includes hypoxemic patients without underlying chronic lung disease and without cardiogenic pulmonary edema. The main reason for acute hypoxemic respiratory failure in nearly three-quarters of the cases is pneumonia, and hypercapnia is uncommon [1–4].

J.-P. Frat (✉) · D. Marie
CHU de Poitiers, Médecine Intensive Réanimation, Poitiers, France

Université de Poitiers, Faculté de Médecine et de Pharmacie de Poitiers, Poitiers, France

INSERM, CIC-1402, équipe 5 ALIVE, Poitiers, France
e-mail: jean-pierre.frat@chu-poitiers.fr

J. Messika
Assistance Publique des Hôpitaux de Paris, Hôpital Bichat, Service de Pneumologie B et Transplantation pulmonaire, Paris, France

Université Paris Diderot, UMR PHERE 1152, Sorbonne Paris Cité, Paris, France

INSERM, PHERE 1152, Paris, France

J.-D. Ricard
Assistance Publique des Hôpitaux de Paris, Hôpital Louis Mourier, Service de Réanimation Médico-Chirurgicale, Colombes, France

Université Paris Diderot, UMR IAME 1137, Sorbonne Paris Cité, Paris, France

INSERM, IAME 1137, Paris, France

© Springer Nature Switzerland AG 2021
A. Carlucci, S. M. Maggiore (eds.), *High Flow Nasal Cannula*,
https://doi.org/10.1007/978-3-030-42454-1_4

Oxygen therapy delivered via face mask with reservoir bag has long been the first-line therapy of choice in acute respiratory failure. However, this strategy has many limits and fails to provide ventilatory support or reduce work of breathing. The fraction of inspired oxygen (FiO2) delivered is limited [5] and comfort is compromised by dry gas [6], which may also impair mucociliary clearance. High-flow nasal cannula oxygen therapy (HFNC) is currently spreading in adult ICU after first being used in preterm neonates and pediatric care, as a first-line treatment for respiratory distress syndrome, and apnea of prematurity. Paradoxically, clinical benefits of HFNC [3, 4, 7] have been first described before understanding its physiological mechanisms. More recently, physiological, pilot studies and controlled trials have drawn attention to HFNC's potential role in adults. HFNC is a strategy providing good comfort through warmed and humidified gas flow delivered via nasal prongs. It preserves high FiO_2 [5] and generates a low level of positive pressure in the upper airways due to a high flow of gas [8], which also provides washout of dead space in the upper airways [9]. Physiological effects of HFNC may help to improve gas exchange and to decrease work of breathing through reducing respiratory rate, proportionally to gas flow, without increased risk of barotrauma [10, 11].

In this chapter we focus on HFNC's clinical applications during acute hypoxemic respiratory failure.

4.2   Patients with Acute Hypoxemic Respiratory Failure

Many oxygen delivery strategies are available in intensive care units including standard oxygen through face mask, NIV, or HFNC. Table 4.1 shows the main randomized controlled trials comparing HFNC with other oxygen delivery techniques in acute respiratory failure. A randomized controlled trial (FLORALI study) reported in 2015 by Frat and colleagues compared these three strategies of oxygenation: standard oxygen, HFNC alone, and NIV interspaced with HFNC [3]. A total of 310 non-hypercapnic patients were included with acute hypoxemic respiratory failure defined by a respiratory rate above 25 breaths per minute, a PaO2/FiO2 < 300 mm Hg, and a PaCO2 ≤ 45 mmHg [3]. The mortality rate at day 90 was lower with HFNC than using the other two strategies: 12% with HFNC versus 23% with standard oxygen and 28% with NIV, $p = 0.02$. Although the rate of intubation was not significantly different among the three groups in the overall population, it was significantly lower among the severe hypoxemic patients (PaO2/FiO2 ≤ 200 mmHg) treated with HFNC than in those treated with oxygen or NIV (35%, 53%, and 58%, respectively, $p = 0.009$). One hour after initiation of HFNC, the dyspnea score and discomfort felt by the patients were significantly lower as compared to standard oxygen or NIV. This study highlighted the deleterious effect of NIV, in terms of risk of mortality and intubation especially in patients with severe acute hypoxemic respiratory failure, and provided for the first time strong evidence on the benefits of HFNC suggested earlier in observational studies [4, 7].

The use of NIV remains debated in patients with acute hypoxemic respiratory failure, and recent European/American clinical practice guidelines were unable to

Table 4.1 Main randomized controlled trials comparing HFNC with other oxygen delivery techniques in acute respiratory failure

Study reference, year, setting	Number of patients, population	Initial settings: HFNC (flow, FiO_2) O_2 (flow)	Intubation rate or escalation in ventilation therapy	Mortality
Frat, 2015 [3], intensive care unit	**$N = 313$** **Inclusion**: RR > 25 breaths/min, $PaO_2/FiO_2 \leq 300$, on ≥ 10 L/min O_2 **Exclusion**: Asthma, chronic lung diseases, hypercapnia, cardiogenic pulmonary edema	**HFNC** 50 L/min, 100% **Non-rebreathing mask** ≥ 10 L/min	**Intubation rate** HFNC: 38% O_2: 47% NIV: 50%	**90 days** HFNC: 12% O_2: 23% NIV: 28%
Azoulay, 2018 [12], intensive care unit	**$N = 778$** **Inclusion**: PaO_2 < 60 mmHg or SpO_2 < 90% on room air or respiratory distress, ≥ 6 L/min O2, immunosuppression **Exclusion**: Hypercapnia, cardiogenic pulmonary edema, recent surgery	**HFNC** 50 L/min, 100% **Nasal prongs or mask** Flow set for $SpO_2 \geq 95\%$	**Intubation rate** HFNC: 39% O_2: 44%	**28 days** HFNC: 36% O_2: 36%
Frat, 2016 [13], intensive care unit (post hoc analysis)	**$N = 82$** **Inclusion**: RR > 25 breaths/min, $PaO_2/FiO_2 \leq 300$, on ≥ 10 L/min O_2, immunosuppression **Exclusion**: Asthma, chronic lung diseases, hypercapnia, cardiogenic pulmonary edema	**HFNC** 50 L/min, 100% **Non-rebreathing mask** ≥ 10 L/min	**Intubation rate** HFNC: 31% O_2: 43% NIV: 65%	**90 days** HFNC: 15% O_2: 27% NIV: 46%
Bell, 2015 [14], emergency department	**$N = 100$** **Inclusion**: RR ≥ 25 breaths/min, $SpO_2 \leq 93\%$ **Exclusion**: Urgent indication of NIV or intubation	**HFNC** 50 L/min, 30% **Nasal prongs or face mask** NA	**Escalation in ventilation therapy** HFNC: 4% O_2: 19%	NA
Jones, 2016 [15], emergency department	**$N = 322$** **Inclusion**: $SpO_2 \leq 92\%$ on room air, RR ≥ 22 breaths/min **Exclusion**: Urgent indication of NIV or intubation	**HFNC** 40 L/min, 28% **Nasal prongs or face mask** NA	**Intubation rate** HFNC: 6% O_2: 12%	**In-hospital** HFNC: 9% O_2: 8%

(continued)

Table 4.1 (continued)

Study reference, year, setting	Number of patients, population	Initial settings: HFNC (flow, FiO$_2$) O$_2$ (flow)	Intubation rate or escalation in ventilation therapy	Mortality
Makdee, 2017 [16], emergency department	**N = 136** **Inclusion**: Cardiogenic pulmonary edema, SpO$_2$ < 95% on Room air, RR >24 breaths/min **Exclusion**: Urgent indication of NIV or intubation, hemodynamic instability, RR >35 breaths/min, SpO$_2$ < 90%, end-stage renal disease	**HFNC** 35 L/min, NA **Nasal prongs or face mask** NA	**Escalation in ventilation therapy** HFNC: 3% O$_2$: 5%	**7 days** HFNC: 2% O$_2$: 0%
Rittayamai, 2015 [17], emergency department	**N = 40** **Inclusion**: RR > 24 breaths/min, SpO2 < 94% on room air **Exclusion**: Urgent intubation, CV instability, chronic respiratory failure	**HFNC** 35 L/min, NA **Nasal prongs or face mask** NA	**Escalation in ventilation therapy** HFNC: 0% O$_2$: 0%	NA

HFNC high-flow nasal cannula oxygen therapy, *NIV* noninvasive ventilation, *RR* respiratory rate, *NA* not available

offer a recommendation given the uncertainty of evidence [18]. The rates of intubation are particularly high in these patients, ranging from 30% to 60%, and although NIV may decrease the risk of intubation as compared with standard oxygen, no significant difference was found in terms of mortality by pooling all randomized controlled trials [3, 19–27].

Although mechanical ventilation either invasive or noninvasive is needed to meet the criteria for acute respiratory syndrome (ARDS) according to the Berlin definition [28], several recent studies have suggested that ARDS might be considered early in patients breathing spontaneously without mechanical ventilation [29]. In a recent study analyzing 127 patients with pulmonary bilateral infiltrates and a PaO$_2$/FiO$_2$ ratio ≤ 300 mm Hg under standard oxygen and then treated by NIV, 120 (94%) fulfilled the criteria for ARDS once NIV was initiated, meaning that these patients could be identified early under standard oxygen in the emergency room [29]. Another study has compared biomarker levels of inflammation and injury in hypoxemic patients with pulmonary bilateral infiltrates either breathing spontaneously or under mechanical ventilation [30]. After propensity score-matched analysis including 39 patients treated with HFNC and 39 intubated patients with usual criteria for ARDS, the pattern for biomarkers of inflammation and injury was similar between the two groups.

Considering patients with acute hypoxemic respiratory failure at risk of ARDS facilitates the understanding of the potential deleterious effect of NIV in patients with acute hypoxemic respiratory failure. A recent sub-analysis of the FLORALI study found that a tidal volume exceeding 9 mL/kg of predicted body weight after 1 h of NIV was a strong factor associated with intubation and mortality [31]. In contrast, time to intubation was not significantly different between survivors and non-survivors, a finding suggesting that poor outcomes were not due to delayed intubation. Moreover, pressure support levels did not differ between patients who needed intubation and the others, and high tidal volumes were probably the consequence of a high patient inspiratory effort [32]. Whereas this may reflect a higher severity of the respiratory disease, patients receiving HFNC with NIV had higher mortality than those receiving HFNC alone, a finding suggesting that pressure support may worsen outcome [3]. An observational study had previously reported that patients treated with NIV for acute hypoxemic respiratory failure and generating a tidal volume above 9.5 ml/kg had an increased risk of intubation as compared with the others [16]. In this study, nearly half of the patients generated tidal volumes above 10 ml/kg despite a target of tidal volume between 6 and 8 ml/kg. Likewise, a recent propensity-matched analysis from a large cohort study focusing on patients with ARDS found that patients with PaO_2/FIO_2 lower than 150 mm Hg and treated with NIV had higher in-ICU mortality than those intubated without prior NIV [15]. These recent studies suggest that NIV may be associated with an increased risk of mortality, and that it should be cautiously used in patients with acute hypoxemic respiratory failure. Ventilator-induced lung injury is well demonstrated in intubated patients under invasive mechanical ventilation and reduction in tidal volumes has clearly decreased mortality in ARDS patients [17]. Surprisingly, tidal volumes generated under NIV have never been mentioned in previous studies [19–27], suggesting that until recently, lung injury potentially induced by NIV had not been considered.

The concept of patient self-inflicted lung injury (P-SILI) developed in recent reviews can explain limits of standard oxygen during the management of patients with acute hypoxemic respiratory failure [14, 16]. It suggests that patients with acute hypoxemic respiratory failure who breathe spontaneously under standard oxygen may worsen their lung injury by generating large efforts, high tidal volumes, and subsequent high transpulmonary pressures, promoting capillary leak and lung edema [14, 16]. Indeed, as compared to standard oxygen HFNC seems to be more beneficial, although patients breathe spontaneously [3]. The physiological effects of HFNC (described in another chapter) especially the low level of positive pressure generated in airways [8, 33, 34] and the washout of upper airways [9] that lead to a decrease in inspiratory effort improve respiratory conditions and may ensure prevention of lung injury (P-SILI).

Therefore, HFNC seems to be a good alternative to standard oxygen in the management of patients with acute hypoxemic respiratory failure, where NIV is no longer recommended [35]. An algorithm summarizing the management of patients with acute respiratory failure is reported in Fig. 4.1.

Fig. 4.1 Algorithm
summarizing the
management of patients
with acute respiratory
failure

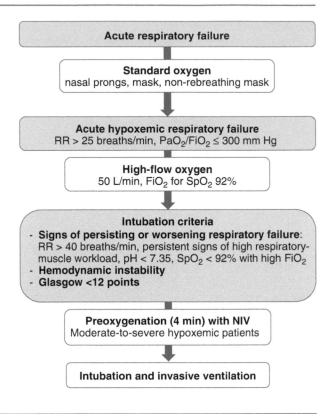

4.3   How to Predict Outcome of HFNC

Because delaying intubation in patients with persistent respiratory distress may worsen their outcome, physicians' concern when initiating HFNC should be to correctly identify those patients that will require intubation and in a timely fashion. The risks of pursuing noninvasive ventilatory support during acute hypoxemic respiratory failure have been clearly identified during both NIV [36] and HFNC [13, 37] and show an increased mortality when intubation occurs after 48 hours. Efforts have thus been made to try to predict success or failure of HFNC. Patients under HFNC should be closely monitored in order to detect signs of failure. This assessment relies on various parameters: first, the clinical signs of respiratory failure; next, the presence of an additional organ failure, apart from respiratory; last, the radiological aspect.

Signs of respiratory failure have been assessed either separately [4, 31] or in association [38, 39]. Sztrymf et al. [4] showed, in a prospective cohort of 38 patients with respiratory failure treated with HFNC, that those patients who required intubation maintained a high respiratory rate and persistent thoracoabdominal asynchrony in comparison with those who succeeded. Oxygenation was also better in patients with HFNC success [4]. Roca et al. [38] created an index, named ROX for "Respiratory rate-OXygenation," aiming to predict the risk for subsequent intubation. The ROX index is defined as the ratio of pulse oximetry/fraction of inspired oxygen to respiratory rate. The ROX index was calculated in 157 patients with pneumonia initially treated with HFNC. It showed the best prediction accuracy when performed 12 h after the onset of HFNC treatment, with a best cutoff point of 4.88, with a ROX index >4.88 at 12 h being predictive of a lower risk of HFNC failure (HR 0.273 [0.121–0.618]; $p = 0.002$). This 4.88 threshold was validated in a prospective cohort of 191 pneumonia patients [39]. Interestingly, the prediction accuracy of this cutoff increased over time. It significantly predicted the success of HFNC as early as 2 h of HFNC onset, with a significantly higher performance at 12 h. In addition, a ROX index below 3.85 at 12 h after HFNC initiation was significantly associated with a risk of HFNC failure. An interesting feature of the ROX index is its dynamic over time: patients whose index did not increase over time were more at risk of intubation than those in whom the value of the index increased over the first 12 h. Dyspnea and respiratory discomfort should be carefully monitored. It has been shown, in a post hoc analysis of the FLORALI trial [31], that respiratory discomfort, assessed after 1 h of HFNC by a visual analogic scale, was lower in patients who succeeded the HFNC strategy (25 ± 23 vs. 36 ± 29).

As it has been shown for NIV [12], the presence of an additional organ failure, other than respiratory, should refrain to pursue HFNC therapy. In a monocenter series of 51 ARDS patients treated with HFNC as first step [40], factors significantly associated with HFNC failure were a higher severity (attested by the Simplified Acute Physiologic Score II) and the occurrence of an additional organ failure. Similar findings have been reported by Koga et al. [41], as a greater SOFA score had been evidenced in patients failing HFNC. In a similar manner, the increase of heart rate after 1 h of HFNC has been reported to be significantly associated with intubation [31].

Last, the radiological aspect should be taken into account and the object of physicians' attention. Indeed, Koga et al. [41] reported that the abundance of pleural effusion, evaluated by chest radiographs, was independently associated with HFNC failure, whereas the number of quadrant opacities did not differ according to the success of the strategy.

To summarize, it should be emphasized that the assessment of patients with HFNC for hypoxemic ARF should encompass a clinical approach, with the repeated calculation of the ROX index and the careful detection of an additional organ failure and a radiological one.

4.4   Patients Admitted in the ED for Acute Respiratory Failure

Previous studies conducted in the emergency departments compared HFNC with standard oxygen in heterogeneous populations of patients with acute respiratory failure due to pneumonia, cardiogenic pulmonary edema, and COPD exacerbation [42–44]. Results were mainly changes in physiological parameters including the reduction of dyspnea and an increase of oxygenation under HFNC [42–44]. One randomized study including 128 patients having cardiogenic pulmonary edema showed a more rapid decrease in respiratory rate within the first 15 minutes of treatment with HFNC as compared to conventional oxygen [45]. Another randomized controlled study compared HFOT with NIV in 204 patients requiring NIV mainly for COPD exacerbation (39% of patients) [46]. HFNC was noninferior to NIV as concerned need for intubation and decision to apply alternate therapy [46].

Consequently, HFOT seems to be an alternative to standard oxygen as first-line therapy to manage patients with acute respiratory failure in the ED. However, NIV remains the recommended treatment for cardiogenic pulmonary edema and COPD exacerbation with respiratory acidosis [18] and HFOT may be applied as an alternate treatment in case of NIV intolerance.

4.5   Immunocompromised Patients with Acute Respiratory Failure

Recent European/American guidelines recommend early NIV for immunocompromised patients with acute respiratory failure [18]. As the need for intubation is associated with particularly high mortality rate in this subset of patients, even more aggressive noninvasive strategies than in non-immunocompromised patients were assessed to avoid intubation. In the early 2000s, two randomized controlled trials reported lower intubation rates and mortality with NIV than with standard oxygen [47, 48]. However, the largest randomized controlled trial carried out to date, including 374 patients, did not confirm potential benefits of NIV, and found similar outcomes in immunocompromised patients with acute respiratory failure treated with NIV or with oxygen alone [49].

Other studies focusing only on immunocompromised patients found better outcomes with high-flow oxygen therapy alone than with NIV [50, 51], thereby suggesting potential deleterious effects of NIV even in immunocompromised patients. Application of high-flow oxygen therapy has been increasing and in a prospective international observational study focusing on immunocompromised patients, the first-line strategy of oxygenation was standard oxygen in 54% of the patients, NIV in 26%, and high-flow oxygen therapy in 20% [52]. After adjustment, high-flow oxygen therapy was associated with a decreased risk of intubation without effect on mortality, whereas NIV had no impact on intubation or mortality.

However, a large randomized controlled trial reported recently by Azoulay and colleagues comparing standard oxygen with HFNC in immunocompromised patients having acute respiratory failure found no difference in terms of mortality and intubation rates between these two strategies [53]. Mortality rates at day 28 were 36% in patients treated with HFNC and treated with standard oxygen ($p = 0.94$). Although this trial was the largest ever conducted in this setting, it did not answer properly the question on the superiority of HFNC versus standard oxygen. Indeed, the calculation of mortality rates had included patients died after intubation due to oxygen strategies' failure, but also patients who died without being intubated because of a "non-full code management." This may have mitigated the positive effect of treatment and increased the mortality in groups of treatment. Considering the mortality rates including all cases of death interferes with the interpretation of results as the efficacy of oxygenation strategies was not the objective in more than one-third of patients.

Studies showed that NIV could be deleterious or at best as efficient as standard oxygen, and that HFNC provided no benefits as compared to standard oxygen. However, NIV remains the most common strategy for these patients, and future studies should confirm the place of HFNC in the management of immunocompromised patients with acute respiratory failure: HFNC with NIV sessions versus high-flow oxygen therapy alone.

4.6   NIV for Preoxygenation of Hypoxemic Patients

Severe oxygen desaturation, usually defined as a drop in peripheral oxygen saturation (SpO_2) below 80%, occurs in 20–25% of intubations in the ICU [54, 55]. Preoxygenation before intubation could prevent oxygen desaturation and the subsequent risk of cardiac arrest, which can occur in 2–3% of the cases [56]. However, the best strategy of preoxygenation has not been clearly established.

NIV and HFNC are two oxygenation devices largely used in ICU that provide higher fraction of inspired oxygen (FIO2) than standard oxygen [3, 5, 57, 58]. HFNC enables delivery of continuous high gas flow via nasal prongs resulting in higher FiO_2 than with standard oxygen [5]. Another theoretical advantage of HFNC may consist of maintaining oxygenation during the apneic phase of intubation after anesthetic induction, thereby avoiding hypoxemia whereas noninvasive ventilation is removed at this phase [59].

One randomized controlled study including a small sample of patients has found a lower incidence of severe oxygen desaturation using NIV as compared to standard bag-valve-mask before intubation in ICU [60]. A larger trial including 201 patients failed to demonstrate any benefits of NIV as a preoxygenation method to reduce organ dysfunction compared with standard bag-valve-mask [61]. However, in patients treated by NIV prior to preoxygenation, there was a higher incidence of severe oxygen desaturation in case of preoxygenation with standard oxygen, suggesting that NIV should probably not be discontinued for preoxygenation in patients treated by NIV before intubation.

A prospective before-after study reported a decrease in episodes of severe oxygen desaturation using HFNC as preoxygenation rather than standard oxygen [62]. These encouraging results were confirmed in a very recent randomized controlled trial comparing HFNC to bag-valve-mask oxygenation (BVM) [63]. Although the median lowest SpO_2 was similar in both groups, mild desaturation below 95% was significantly more frequent with BVM (23%) than with HFNC (12%). There were significantly fewer adverse events in the HFNC group than in the BVM group, including fewer severe adverse events. These positive results are in agreement with several meta-analyses that have consistently showed that preoxygenation with HFNC was superior to standard bag-valve-mask [64, 65].

A recent multicenter randomized controlled trial (FLORALI-2 study) comparing NIV and HFNC for preoxygenation in 313 hypoxemic patients undergoing intubation was recently reported [66, 67]. Preoxygenation with noninvasive ventilation as compared with HFNC did not change the risk of severe hypoxemia during intubation procedure or the occurrence of late complications *(The Lancet Respiratory Medicine in press)*. However, baseline PaO_2:FiO_2 ratio appeared to modify the effect of preoxygenation strategies on the risk of severe hypoxemia, with secondary analyses suggesting a possible benefit of noninvasive ventilation among patients with moderate-to-severe hypoxemia. Noninvasive ventilation may prevent severe hypoxemia among patients with severe-moderate hypoxemia (PaO_2:$FiO_2 \leq 200$ mmHg) as compared with high-flow oxygen. This finding calls for confirmation in future research.

4.7   Remaining Questions

The superiority of HFNC in patients with acute hypoxemic respiratory failure on other oxygen delivery techniques, i.e., NIV and standard oxygen, has been reported in only one randomized controlled trial. Benefits of HFNC were markedly more significant in the subgroup of severe hypoxemic patients. Surprisingly, these results were not reproducible in immunocompromised patients when HFNC was compared with standard oxygen, while NIV was not superior to standard oxygen in this setting. Moreover, the application of NIV as first-line therapy was not retained by recent guidelines on acute hypoxemic respiratory failure. Therefore, future studies should compare HFNC with standard oxygen in acute hypoxemic respiratory failure, to confirm the potential superiority of HFNC.

4.8   Conclusion

Recent studies have led to applying of HFNC in place of standard oxygen in patients with acute hypoxemic respiratory failure; however in immunocompromised patients, standard oxygen appeared to be as efficient as HFNC. This calls for future studies to define the place of HFNC. When patients fail a noninvasive strategy, those with severe hypoxemia should be preoxygenated rather with NIV than with HFNC, whereas those with mild hypoxemia can be preoxygenated with HFNC.

References

1. Contou D, Fragnoli C, Córdoba-Izquierdo A, Boissier F, Brun-Buisson C, Thille AW. Noninvasive ventilation for acute hypercapnic respiratory failure: intubation rate in an experienced unit. Respir Care. 2013;58(12):2045–52.
2. Thille AW, Contou D, Fragnoli C, Cordoba-Izquierdo A, Boissier F, Brun-Buisson C. Noninvasive ventilation for acute hypoxemic respiratory failure: intubation rate and risk factors. Crit Care. 2013;17(6):R269. Pubmed Central PMCID: PMC4057073. Epub 2013/11/13. eng

3. Frat JP, Thille AW, Mercat A, Girault C, Ragot S, Perbet S, et al. High-flow oxygen through nasal cannula in acute hypoxemic respiratory failure. N Engl J Med. 2015;372(23):2185–96. Epub 2015/05/20. eng
4. Sztrymf B, Messika J, Bertrand F, Hurel D, Leon R, Dreyfuss D, et al. Beneficial effects of humidified high flow nasal oxygen in critical care patients: a prospective pilot study. Intensive Care Med. 2011;37(11):1780–6.
5. Sim MA, Dean P, Kinsella J, Black R, Carter R, Hughes M. Performance of oxygen delivery devices when the breathing pattern of respiratory failure is simulated. Anaesthesia. 2008;63(9):938–40.
6. Roca O, Riera J, Torres F, Masclans JR. High-flow oxygen therapy in acute respiratory failure. Respir Care. 2010;55(4):408–13.
7. Sztrymf B, Messika J, Mayot T, Lenglet H, Dreyfuss D, Ricard JD. Impact of high-flow nasal cannula oxygen therapy on intensive care unit patients with acute respiratory failure: a prospective observational study. J Crit Care. 2012;27(3):324. e9–13
8. Parke R, McGuinness S, Eccleston M. Nasal high-flow therapy delivers low level positive airway pressure. Br J Anaesth. 2009;103(6):886–90. Pubmed Central PMCID: PMC2777940. Epub 2009/10/23. eng
9. Moller W, Feng S, Domanski U, Franke KJ, Celik G, Bartenstein P, et al. Nasal high flow reduces dead space. J Appl Physiol (Bethesda, Md : 1985). 2017;122(1):191–7. Pubmed Central PMCID: PMC5283847. Epub 2016/11/20. eng
10. Mauri T, Turrini C, Eronia N, Grasselli G, Volta CA, Bellani G, et al. Physiologic effects of high-flow nasal cannula in acute hypoxemic respiratory failure. Am J Respir Crit Care Med. 2017;195(9):1207–15. Epub 2016/12/21. eng
11. Delorme M, Bouchard PA, Simon M, Simard S, Lellouche F. Effects of high-flow nasal cannula on the work of breathing in patients recovering from acute respiratory failure. Crit Care Med. 2017;45(12):1981–8. Epub 2017/09/01. eng
12. Antonelli M, Conti G, Esquinas A, Montini L, Maggiore SM, Bello G, et al. A multiple-center survey on the use in clinical practice of noninvasive ventilation as a first-line intervention for acute respiratory distress syndrome. Crit Care Med. 2007;35(1):18–25. Epub 2006/11/30. eng
13. Kang BJ, Koh Y, Lim CM, Huh JW, Baek S, Han M, et al. Failure of high-flow nasal cannula therapy may delay intubation and increase mortality. Intensive Care Med. 2015;41(4):623–32. Epub 2015/02/19. eng
14. Brochard L. Ventilation-induced lung injury exists in spontaneously breathing patients with acute respiratory failure: yes. Intensive Care Med. 2017;43(2):250–2. Epub 2017/01/12. eng
15. Bellani G, Laffey JG, Pham T, Madotto F, Fan E, Brochard L, et al. Noninvasive ventilation of patients with acute respiratory distress syndrome. Insights from the LUNG SAFE study. Am J Respir Crit Care Med. 2017;195(1):67–77. Epub 2016/10/19. eng
16. Brochard L, Slutsky A, Pesenti A. Mechanical ventilation to minimize progression of lung injury in acute respiratory failure. Am J Respir Crit Care Med. 2017;195(4):438–42. Epub 2016/09/15. eng
17. Ventilation with lower tidal volumes as compared with traditional tidal volumes for acute lung injury and the acute respiratory distress syndrome. The acute respiratory distress syndrome network. N Engl J Med. 2000;342(18):1301–8. Epub 2000/05/04. eng
18. Rochwerg B, Brochard L, Elliott MW, Hess D, Hill NS, Nava S, et al. Official ERS/ATS clinical practice guidelines: noninvasive ventilation for acute respiratory failure. Eur Respir J. 2017;50:2. Pubmed Central PMCID: PMC5593345 erj.ersjournals.com. Epub 2017/09/02. eng
19. Antonelli M, Conti G, Rocco M, Bufi M, De Blasi RA, Vivino G, et al. A comparison of non-invasive positive-pressure ventilation and conventional mechanical ventilation in patients with acute respiratory failure. N Engl J Med. 1998;339(7):429–35. Epub 1998/08/13. eng
20. Ferrer M, Esquinas A, Leon M, Gonzalez G, Alarcon A, Torres A. Noninvasive ventilation in severe hypoxemic respiratory failure: a randomized clinical trial. Am J Respir Crit Care Med. 2003;168(12):1438–44. Epub 2003/09/23. eng

21. Confalonieri M, Potena A, Carbone G, Porta RD, Tolley EA, Umberto MG. Acute respiratory failure in patients with severe community-acquired pneumonia. A prospective randomized evaluation of noninvasive ventilation. Am J Respir Crit Care Med. 1999;160(5 Pt 1):1585–91. Epub 1999/11/11. eng
22. Martin TJ, Hovis JD, Costantino JP, Bierman MI, Donahoe MP, Rogers RM, et al. A randomized, prospective evaluation of noninvasive ventilation for acute respiratory failure. Am J Respir Crit Care Med. 2000;161(3 Pt 1):807–13. Epub 2000/03/11. eng
23. Wysocki M, Tric L, Wolff MA, Millet H, Herman B. Noninvasive pressure support ventilation in patients with acute respiratory failure. A randomized comparison with conventional therapy. Chest. 1995;107(3):761–8. Epub 1995/03/01. eng
24. Honrubia T, Garcia Lopez FJ, Franco N, Mas M, Guevara M, Daguerre M, et al. Noninvasive vs conventional mechanical ventilation in acute respiratory failure: a multicenter, randomized controlled trial. Chest. 2005;128(6):3916–24. Epub 2005/12/16. eng
25. Zhan Q, Sun B, Liang L, Yan X, Zhang L, Yang J, et al. Early use of noninvasive positive pressure ventilation for acute lung injury: a multicenter randomized controlled trial. Crit Care Med. 2012;40(2):455–60. Epub 2011/10/25. eng
26. Kramer N, Meyer TJ, Meharg J, Cece RD, Hill NS. Randomized, prospective trial of noninvasive positive pressure ventilation in acute respiratory failure. Am J Respir Crit Care Med. 1995;151(6):1799–806. Epub 1995/06/01. eng
27. Wood KA, Lewis L, Von Harz B, Kollef MH. The use of noninvasive positive pressure ventilation in the emergency department: results of a randomized clinical trial. Chest. 1998;113(5):1339–46. Epub 1998/05/22. eng
28. Ranieri VM, Rubenfeld GD, Thompson BT, Ferguson ND, Caldwell E, Fan E, et al. Acute respiratory distress syndrome: the Berlin definition. JAMA. 2012;307(23):2526–33.
29. Coudroy R, Frat JP, Boissier F, Contou D, Robert R, Thille AW. Early identification of acute respiratory distress syndrome in the absence of positive pressure ventilation: implications for revision of the Berlin criteria for acute respiratory distress syndrome. Crit Care Med. 2018;46(4):540–6. Epub 2017/12/23. eng
30. Garcia-de-Acilu M, Marin-Corral J, Vazquez A, Ruano L, Magret M, Ferrer R, et al. Hypoxemic patients with bilateral infiltrates treated with high-flow nasal cannula present a similar pattern of biomarkers of inflammation and injury to acute respiratory distress syndrome patients. Crit Care Med. 2017;45(11):1845–53. Epub 2017/08/15. eng
31. Frat JP, Ragot S, Coudroy R, Constantin JM, Girault C, Prat G, et al. Predictors of intubation in patients with acute hypoxemic respiratory failure treated with a noninvasive oxygenation strategy. Crit Care Med. 2018;46(2):208–15. Epub 2017/11/04. eng
32. Carteaux G, Millan-Guilarte T, De Prost N, Razazi K, Abid S, Thille AW, et al. Failure of noninvasive ventilation for De novo acute hypoxemic respiratory failure: role of tidal volume. Crit Care Med. 2016;44(2):282–90. Epub 2015/11/20. eng
33. Parke RL, Bloch A, McGuinness SP. Effect of very-high-flow nasal therapy on airway pressure and end-expiratory lung impedance in healthy volunteers. Respir Care. 2015;60(10):1397–403. Epub 2015/09/04. eng
34. Parke RL, Eccleston ML, McGuinness SP. The effects of flow on airway pressure during nasal high-flow oxygen therapy. Respir Care. 2011;56(8):1151–5.
35. Rochwerg B, Einav S, Chaudhuri D, Mancebo J, Mauri T, Helviz Y, et al. The role for high flow nasal cannula as a respiratory support strategy in adults: a clinical practice guideline. Intensive Care Med. 2020;46(12):2226–37.
36. Carrillo A, Gonzalez-Diaz G, Ferrer M, Martinez-Quintana ME, Lopez-Martinez A, Llamas N, et al. Non-invasive ventilation in community-acquired pneumonia and severe acute respiratory failure. Intensive Care Med. 2012;38(3):458–66.
37. Ricard JD, Messika J, Sztrymf B, Gaudry S. Impact on outcome of delayed intubation with high-flow nasal cannula oxygen: is the device solely responsible? Intensive Care Med. 2015;41(6):1157–8. Epub 2015/04/15. eng
38. Roca O, Messika J, Caralt B, Garcia-de-Acilu M, Sztrymf B, Ricard JD, et al. Predicting success of high-flow nasal cannula in pneumonia patients with hypoxemic respiratory failure: the utility of the ROX index. J Crit Care. 2016;35:200–5. Epub 2016/08/03. eng

39. Roca O, Caralt B, Messika J, Samper M, Sztrymf B, Hernandez G, et al. An index combining respiratory rate and oxygenation to predict outcome of nasal high flow therapy. Am J Respir Crit Care Med. 2018;21. Epub 2018/12/24. eng

40. Messika J, Ben Ahmed K, Gaudry S, Miguel-Montanes R, Rafat C, Sztrymf B, et al. Use of high-flow nasal cannula oxygen therapy in subjects with ARDS: a 1-year observational study. Respir Care. 2015;60(2):162–9. Epub 2014/11/06. eng

41. Koga Y, Kaneda K, Mizuguchi I, Nakahara T, Miyauchi T, Fujita M, et al. Extent of pleural effusion on chest radiograph is associated with failure of high-flow nasal cannula oxygen therapy. J Crit Care. 2016;32:165–9. Epub 2016/01/15. eng

42. Jones PG, Kamona S, Doran O, Sawtell F, Wilsher M. Randomized controlled trial of humidified high-flow nasal oxygen for acute respiratory distress in the emergency department: the HOT-ER study. Respir Care. 2016;61(3):291–9. Epub 2015/11/19. eng

43. Rittayamai N, Tscheikuna J, Praphruetkit N, Kijpinyochai S. Use of high-flow nasal cannula for acute Dyspnea and hypoxemia in the emergency department. Respir Care. 2015;60(10):1377–82. Epub 2015/06/11. eng

44. Bell N, Hutchinson CL, Green TC, Rogan E, Bein KJ, Dinh MM. Randomised control trial of humidified high flow nasal cannulae versus standard oxygen in the emergency department. Emerg Med Australas. 2015;27(6):537–41. Epub 2015/10/01. eng

45. Makdee O, Monsomboon A, Surabenjawong U, Praphruetkit N, Chaisirin W, Chakorn T, et al. High-flow nasal cannula versus conventional oxygen therapy in emergency department patients with cardiogenic pulmonary Edema: a randomized controlled trial. Ann Emerg Med. 2017;70(4):465–72. e2. Epub 2017/06/12. eng

46. Doshi P, Whittle JS, Bublewicz M, Kearney J, Ashe T, Graham R, et al. High-velocity nasal insufflation in the treatment of respiratory failure: a randomized clinical trial. Ann Emerg Med. 2018;5. Epub 2018/01/10. eng

47. Antonelli M, Conti G, Bufi M, Costa MG, Lappa A, Rocco M, et al. Noninvasive ventilation for treatment of acute respiratory failure in patients undergoing solid organ transplantation: a randomized trial. JAMA. 2000;283(2):235–41.

48. Hilbert G, Gruson D, Vargas F, Valentino R, Gbikpi-Benissan G, Dupon M, et al. Noninvasive ventilation in immunosuppressed patients with pulmonary infiltrates, fever, and acute respiratory failure. N Engl J Med. 2001;344(7):481–7. Epub 2001/02/15. eng

49. Lemiale V, Mokart D, Resche-Rigon M, Pene F, Mayaux J, Faucher E, et al. Effect of noninvasive ventilation vs oxygen therapy on mortality among immunocompromised patients with acute respiratory failure: a randomized clinical trial. JAMA. 2015;314(16):1711–9. Epub 2015/10/08. eng

50. Frat JP, Ragot S, Girault C, Perbet S, Prat G, Boulain T, et al. Effect of non-invasive oxygenation strategies in immunocompromised patients with severe acute respiratory failure: a post-hoc analysis of a randomised trial. Lancet Respir Med. 2016;4(8):646–52. Epub 2016/06/02. eng

51. Coudroy R, Jamet A, Petua P, Robert R, Frat JP, Thille AW. High-flow nasal cannula oxygen therapy versus noninvasive ventilation in immunocompromised patients with acute respiratory failure: an observational cohort study. Ann Intensive Care. 2016;6(1):45. Pubmed Central PMCID: PMC4875575. Epub 2016/05/22. eng

52. Azoulay E, Pickkers P, Soares M, Perner A, Rello J, Bauer PR, et al. Acute hypoxemic respiratory failure in immunocompromised patients: the Efraim multinational prospective cohort study. Intensive Care Med. 2017;43(12):1808–19. Epub 2017/09/28. eng

53. Azoulay E, Lemiale V, Mokart D, Nseir S, Argaud L, Pene F, et al. Effect of high-flow nasal oxygen vs standard oxygen on 28-day mortality in immunocompromised patients with acute respiratory failure: the HIGH randomized clinical trial. JAMA. 2018;24. Epub 2018/10/26. eng

54. Jaber S, Amraoui J, Lefrant JY, Arich C, Cohendy R, Landreau L, et al. Clinical practice and risk factors for immediate complications of endotracheal intubation in the intensive care unit: a prospective, multiple-center study. Crit Care Med. 2006;34(9):2355–61. Epub 2006/07/20. eng

55. Jaber S, Jung B, Corne P, Sebbane M, Muller L, Chanques G, et al. An intervention to decrease complications related to endotracheal intubation in the intensive care unit: a prospective, multiple-center study. Intensive Care Med. 2010;36(2):248–55. Epub 2009/11/19. eng

56. De Jong A, Rolle A, Molinari N, Paugam-Burtz C, Constantin JM, Lefrant JY, et al. Cardiac arrest and mortality related to intubation procedure in critically ill adult patients: a Multicenter cohort study. Crit Care Med. 2018;46(4):532–9. Epub 2017/12/21. eng

57. Frat JP, Brugiere B, Ragot S, Chatellier D, Veinstein A, Goudet V, et al. Sequential application of oxygen therapy via high-flow nasal cannula and noninvasive ventilation in acute respiratory failure: an observational pilot study. Respir Care. 2015;60(2):170–8.

58. L'Her E, Deye N, Lellouche F, Taille S, Demoule A, Fraticelli A, et al. Physiologic effects of non-invasive ventilation during acute lung injury. Am J Respir Crit Care Med. 2005;172(9):1112–8.

59. Ricard JD. Hazards of intubation in the ICU: role of nasal high flow oxygen therapy for preoxygenation and apneic oxygenation to prevent desaturation. Minerva Anestesiol. 2016;82(10):1098–106. Epub 2016/10/18. eng

60. Baillard C, Fosse JP, Sebbane M, Chanques G, Vincent F, Courouble P, et al. Noninvasive ventilation improves preoxygenation before intubation of hypoxic patients. Am J Respir Crit Care Med. 2006;174(2):171–7. Epub 2006/04/22. eng

61. Baillard C, Prat G, Jung B, Futier E, Lefrant JY, Vincent F, et al. Effect of preoxygenation using non-invasive ventilation before intubation on subsequent organ failures in hypoxaemic patients: a randomised clinical trial. Br J Anaesth. 2018;120(2):361–7. Epub 2018/02/07. eng

62. Miguel-Montanes R, Hajage D, Messika J, Bertrand F, Gaudry S, Rafat C, et al. Use of high-flow nasal cannula oxygen therapy to prevent desaturation during tracheal intubation of intensive care patients with mild-to-moderate hypoxemia*. Crit Care Med. 2015;43(3):574–83.

63. Guitton C, Ehrmann S, Volteau C, Colin G, Maamar A, Jean-Michel V, et al. Nasal high-flow preoxygenation for endotracheal intubation in the critically ill patient: a randomized clinical trial. Intensive Care Med. 2019;21. Epub 2019/01/23. eng

64. Tan E, Loubani O, Kureshi N, Green RS. Does apneic oxygenation prevent desaturation during emergency airway management? A systematic review and meta-analysis. Can J Anaesth. 2018;65(8):936–49. Epub 2018/04/25. L'oxygenation apneique previent-elle la desaturation au cours de la gestion des voies respiratoires en urgence? Revue systematique de la litterature et meta-analyse. eng

65. Russotto V, Cortegiani A, Raineri SM, Gregoretti C, Giarratano A. Respiratory support techniques to avoid desaturation in critically ill patients requiring endotracheal intubation: a systematic review and meta-analysis. J Crit Care. 2017;41:98–106. Epub 2017/05/16. eng

66. Frat JP et al. Non-invasive ventilation versus high-flow nasal cannula oxygen therapy with apnoeic oxygenation for preoxygenation before intubation of patients with acute hypoxaemic respiratory failure: a randomised, multicentre, open-label trial. The Lancet Respiratory medicine. 2019;7:303–12

67. Frat JP, Ricard JD, Coudroy R, Robert R, Ragot S, Thille AW. Preoxygenation with non-invasive ventilation versus high-flow nasal cannula oxygen therapy for intubation of patients with acute hypoxaemic respiratory failure in ICU: the prospective randomised controlled FLORALI-2 study protocol. BMJ Open. 2017;7(12):e018611. Pubmed Central PMCID: PMC5770951. Epub 2017/12/25. eng

Clinical Applications of High-Flow Nasal Cannula during Intubation and Weaning from Mechanical Ventilation

5

Mariangela Battilana, Luca Serano,
Carmine Giovanni Iovino, Pierluigi Di Giannatale,
Ivan Dell'Atti, and Salvatore M. Maggiore

5.1 Introduction

Mechanical ventilation is a common procedure in anesthetic practice and critical care medicine. The beginning and the termination of invasive mechanical ventilation are two important phases, which require the placement of an endotracheal tube (intubation) and its successful removal (extubation), respectively.

Although endotracheal intubation is generally a safe procedure, it exposes the patient to the risk of complications, even life-threatening ones, such as severe hypoxemia, dysrhythmia, hemodynamic impairment, cardiac arrest, and death [1, 2]. Preoxygenation before intubation is fundamental for patient safety, as it allows prolonging the time without oxygen desaturation during laryngoscopy, tracheal intubation, or difficult airway management. From a physiological point of view, preoxygenation increases oxygen body reserve through denitrogenation of the lungs, thus extending the safe apnea time, defined as the interval between the apnea onset and the time peripheral capillary oxygen saturation reaches a value $\leq 90\%$. In healthy adults, preoxygenation with 100% FiO_2 prolonged safe apnea time from 1–2 min, in patients breathing room air, to 8 min [1, 3]. An effective preoxygenation is especially important in critically ill patients because several pathological conditions, such as high peripheral oxygen uptake, hemodynamic instability, and altered consciousness, compromise the optimal transfer of oxygen to the lung and the blood [4]. For being effective, preoxygenation requires a methodical approach: end points of maximal

M. Battilana · L. Serano · C. G. Iovino · P. Di Giannatale · I. Dell'Atti
Clinical Department of Anaesthesiology and Intensive Care Medicine,
SS. Annunziata Hospital, Chieti, Italy

S. M. Maggiore (✉)
Clinical Department of Anaesthesiology and Intensive Care Medicine,
SS. Annunziata Hospital, Chieti, Italy

University Department of Innovative Technologies in Medicine & Dentistry, Gabriele d'Annunzio University of Chieti-Pescara, Chieti, Italy
e-mail: salvatore.maggiore@unich.it

© Springer Nature Switzerland AG 2021
A. Carlucci, S. M. Maggiore (eds.), *High Flow Nasal Cannula*,
https://doi.org/10.1007/978-3-030-42454-1_5

preoxygenation efficacy are an end-tidal oxygen concentration of 90% or an end-tidal nitrogen concentration of 5%. The rate of decline in oxyhemoglobin desaturation during apnea time reflects its efficiency [5]. In clinical practice, 3 min is an acceptable duration of preoxygenation for most patients. The most used device for preoxygenation in clinical practice is the non-rebreathing mask. Alternative devices have been proposed to improve the effectiveness of preoxygenation, particularly in emergency and in the critical care setting. For example, noninvasive ventilation (NIV) has been shown to be superior to face mask in terms of preoxygenation effectiveness in hypoxemic patients [6]. HFNC is a more recent device that has been proposed as a tool for preoxygenation either when used alone or in combination with NIV [7].

After preoxygenation, in the period preceding intubation and during the procedure, the patient spends a period of apnea (apneic phase) which can generate an intense hypoxemia that increases the risk of adverse events [8]. During apnea in adults, the rate of oxygen transfer from the alveoli to the blood averages 230 mL/min, whereas carbon dioxide (CO_2) delivery to the alveoli from the venous blood is only 21 mL/min. The result is that lung volume decreases initially by 209 mL/min creating a pressure gradient between the upper airway and the alveoli that allows oxygen passive diffusion if the airways are not obstructed. In the apnea phase, CO_2 cannot be exhaled and the arterial partial pressure of CO_2 ($PaCO_2$) rises to 8–16 mmHg in the first minute of apnea, followed by a linear rise of approximately 3 mmHg/min [5]. Oxygen passive diffusion during apneic phase without manual ventilation, also called *apneic oxygenation*, may be essential to extend the effect of preoxygenation and reduce $PaCO_2$ as a result of the dead-space washout. Apneic oxygenation is therefore recommended in high-risk patients, during emergency intubation, and in anticipated difficult airway management [1]. HFNC may be particularly useful in the apneic phase, even during the insertion of the endotracheal tube, thus allowing a continuous blood oxygenation also when the NIV facial mask or the bag-valve mask (BVM) used for preoxygenation is removed [9–11]. For this reason, several studies focused on the effectiveness of HFNC both for preoxygenation and for apneic ventilation in the operating room (OR) and in the intensive care unit (ICU).

Weaning from mechanical ventilation and removal of the endotracheal tube is a crucial phase of patient management both in postoperative setting and in the ICU. During the transition from mechanical ventilation to unassisted spontaneous breathing, several pathophysiological changes in the airway status and in the cardio-respiratory status may lead to weaning failure and reintubation, especially in high-risk, critically ill patients. Weaning failure results in increased mortality rates (25–50%), prolonged mechanical ventilation, increased incidence of ventilator-associated pneumonia, and longer ICU and hospital stays [12–16]. On the other hand, the unnecessary prolongation of mechanical ventilation also exposes the patient to an increased risk of complications, particularly infectious complications, and increased mortality. Therefore, it is important to identify as soon as possible patients who are ready to start the weaning process and to prevent weaning failure also implementing strategies of ventilatory support after extubation. The available techniques of respiratory support after extubation are conventional oxygen therapy (COT), NIV, and, more recently, HFNC, which has the advantage of being easy to use and generally comfortable for the patient.

5.2   Clinical Application of HFNC during Intubation

5.2.1   HFNC during Intubation Process in Surgical Patients

Several studies have reported the effects of HFNC as a tool for preoxygenation and for apneic oxygenation during intubation in the OR and others are in progress to evaluate its efficacy in different surgical contexts. HFNC has also been assessed in patients at risk for peri-intubation complications, particularly hypoxemia, such as in patients with significant airway and respiratory compromise, during emergency surgery, and in obese patients. However, to date, large randomized trials on the use of HFNC for preoxygenation in the OR are lacking.

Patel and Nouraei described for the first time the use of HFNC in 25 patients with difficult airway management who were undergoing general anesthesia for hypopharyngeal or laryngotracheal surgery, initially to provide preoxygenation, and subsequently to allow apneic oxygenation during intravenous anesthesia and muscular paralysis, until a definitive airway was secured. Reported average apnea time was 17 min, without desaturation and complications suggestive of CO_2 toxicity [17]. Subsequently, Booth et al. reported on the use of HFNC in 30 patients with significant airway and respiratory compromise undergoing general intravenous anesthesia with spontaneous breathing for elective laryngotracheal surgery. This technique, they called STRIVE Hi (SponTaneous Respiration using IntraVEnous anesthesia and Hi-flow nasal oxygen), had several beneficial effects on oxygenation, ventilation, and airway patency. In particular, no case of oxygen saturations below 97%, apnea, or complete airway obstruction was reported. These authors pointed out that patients did not require major upper airway intervention or adjuvant use except for a minor jaw thrust, since high gas flow generates positive airway pressure (Paw) that counteracts the nasopharyngeal structure's collapsibility during anesthesia induction [18].

In a prospective observational study, Doyle et al. found that use of HFNC was associated with a low incidence of desaturation during emergency intubation of patients at high risk of hypoxia in the ICU, OR, and emergency department (ED) [19]. In addition to that, greater comfort has been described by all patients, including those who reported claustrophobia with the standard facial mask. This benefit has also been confirmed in a stressful procedure, such as awake nasal or oral fiberoptic intubation for anticipated difficult airway management [20]. In this study, HFNC was described as the only available method to continuously provide the patient with 100% FiO_2 during the procedure [20]. In another study HFNC was found to be safe and effective for preoxygenation and for maintaining oxygenation in patients receiving rapid sequence induction for urgent/emergency abdominal surgery. This suggests that HFNC is an interesting device for prevention of hypoxemia in emergency, a quite common condition in this setting. In addition, the hemodynamic profile was kept stable throughout the procedure, likely because arterial blood gases were maintained within suitable values [21].

Obese patients are at greater risk for oxygen desaturation during intubation mainly due to the reduction of lung volume available for oxygen storage during the preoxygenation phase and the consequently limited physiologic reserve. A randomized controlled trial, comparing three different preoxygenation procedures prior to rapid sequence induction in morbidly obese patients undergoing bariatric surgery, has shown that PaO_2 at the end of preoxygenation was the highest with HFNC and it was significantly higher than with face mask ($p = 0.048$) [22]. This study suggests that HFNC could provide an effective and safe preoxygenation in obese patients undergoing to general anesthesia.

HFNC is useful during intubation also in children. A recent study reported that apneic oxygenation with HFNC is an easily applied intervention, associated with reduction of hypoxemia during intubation, while nearly 50% of children not receiving apneic oxygenation with this device experienced hypoxemia [23].

A limitation of apneic oxygenation with traditional techniques is the progressive rise in $PaCO_2$. It should be noted, however, that the $PaCO_2$ rise is reduced with HFNC, because of dead-space washout by high flow [24].

Other studies have not shown significant differences between conventional preoxygenation techniques and HFNC, likely because of different settings (i.e., lower gas flow) or patient populations (i.e., sicker patients) [25, 26].

For example, a randomized controlled trial assessed the use of HFNC compared to standard face mask in both preoxygenation and apneic oxygenation in adults who were intubated following a non-rapid sequence induction. After preoxygenation, induction and muscle-relaxant agents were given. Waiting for complete paralysis, patients in the standard face mask group received mask ventilation, whereas patients in the HFNC group received apneic oxygenation with HFNC. No complications were observed in either group. HFNC produced a higher PaO_2 after preoxygenation and safe PaO_2 during intubation. However, the subsequent fall in PaO_2 and rise in $PaCO_2$ indicate that HFNC was not as effective as mask ventilation following neuromuscular blockade [27].

HFNC has been evaluated also for preoxygenation in pregnant women. Tan et al. investigated HFNC using a standardized preoxygenation protocol (30 L min^{-1} for 30 s, then 50 L min^{-1} for 150 s), which resulted to be inadequate to pre-oxygenate pregnant women. The authors discussed that pregnant women may achieve better preoxygenation at higher flows and after a longer time of application than those used in this study. Furthermore, study participants, while actively encouraged to breathe with their mouths closed, were not mandated to do so, decreasing HFNC efficacy on oxygenation and on the level of Paw delivered. In addition, anatomical and physiological changes in pregnancy may change the in vivo aerodynamics of HFNC and decrease the delivered inspired concentration of oxygen and positive airway pressure compared with use in the nonpregnant individual [28].

The Difficult Airway Society guidelines state that the maintenance of adequate oxygenation during advanced airway management is a priority and recommend preoxygenation in all patients before the induction of general anesthesia, since it might prevent desaturation during difficult intubation [3]. A recent study has suggested the systematic implementation of HFNC in the airway control algorithm, as HFNC presents several theoretical advantages compared with the standard face mask, including the ability to deliver continuous oxygen flow during laryngoscopy [2].

Table 5.1 Recommended use of high-flow nasal cannula (HFNC) during intubation and extubation

	Anesthesia	Intensive care unit
Intubation	Suggested use, particularly in patients with anticipated difficult intubation (ability to deliver apneic oxygenation)	Suggested use in patients who are already receiving HFNC, particularly the less severe
Extubation	Suggested use in high-risk and/or obese patients undergoing cardiothoracic surgery	Suggested use in high-risk patients intubated for >24 h

In conclusion, data in the literature suggest that HFNC has potential beneficial effects for preoxygenation and apneic oxygenation in the operating room (Table 5.1). However, other studies are needed to clarify which classes of patients can benefit the most and to standardize its use.

5.2.2   HFNC Clinical Application during Intubation Process in Critically Ill Patients

Critically ill patients are more exposed to procedural adverse effects. A combination of reduced pulmonary functional residual capacity and a compromised cardiovascular reserve may lead to oxygen desaturation, which might occur during tracheal intubation: for this reason, achieving an optimal oxygenation status during intubation is compulsory. Cardiac arrest occurs in 2–3% of intubation procedures in ICU and is strongly associated with hypoxemia or absence of preoxygenation before intubation.

As already mentioned regarding the OR, also in critically ill patients, preoxygenation is performed with reservoir/face mask with an O_2 flow up to 15 L/min or with NIV. NIV showed the ability to reduce adverse events related to intubation in critically ill patients when used for preoxygenation. Baillard et al. compared preoxygenation with NIV with that done with BVM in ICU-admitted hypoxemic patients who required orotracheal intubation. This randomized trial showed that NIV is a more effective device than the standard technique for preoxygenation in this category of patients [6]. HFNC can provide advantages when used for the preparation of the intubation procedure of critically ill patients, particularly because it can be kept in place during laryngoscopy, thus allowing apneic oxygenation and prolongation of the safe apnea time [29, 30].

Several studies have been conducted on the use of HFNC for preoxygenation in the critical care setting. In a subsequent randomized controlled trial including non-severely hypoxemic patients requiring intubation in the ICU, Guitton et al. compared HFNC with standard BVM. Compared with BVM, use of HFNC did not improve the lowest oxygen saturation during intubation but was associated with a reduction in intubation-related adverse events, including severe hypoxemia [4]. In a before-after study, Miguel-Montanes et al. compared non-rebreathing reservoir face mask (NRM) and HFNC for preoxygenation in patients with mild-moderate respiratory failure who were undergoing endotracheal intubation in ICU: the prevalence of desaturation events ($SpO_2 < 80\%$) decreased from 14% in the NRM group to 2% in the HFNC group (p = 0.03) [9]. In 2015, Vourc'h et al. assessed the effects of HFNC during preoxygenation in severely hypoxemic patients requiring orotracheal intubation, as compared with high-FiO_2 facial mask (HFFM). No difference was found in the lowest oxygen saturation throughout the intubation procedure and in the complications rate [25].

Frat et al. have compared NIV with HFNC to assess whether NIV was more efficient than HFNC in reducing the risk of severe hypoxemia during intubation in patients with acute hypoxemic failure. While no significant difference in the incidence of severe hypoxemia and other complications was found, NIV was better in preventing oxygen desaturation during intubation among patients with severe-to-moderate hypoxemia, since the modest PEEP level induced by HFNC and apneic oxygenation alone might not be sufficient to avoid desaturation [31]. The discrepancy between these results is likely due to the different severity of patients enrolled in these studies. HFNC might be more effective in patients with milder hypoxemia, in which the high FiO_2, low PEEP, and apneic oxygenation provided by this device may suffice. In contrast, in studies which enrolled patients with higher degrees of hypoxemia, NIV was shown to give more satisfactory results. In the most hypoxemic patients, Jaber et al. assessed the efficacy of the combined use of HFNC with NIV and showed that HFNC combined with NIV was able to decrease oxygen desaturation during intubation, maintaining higher SpO_2 levels during induction with no severe desaturation ($SpO2 < 80\%$), more than NIV alone, since HFNC provided apneic oxygenation when NIV was removed for the intubation procedure [7].

In a recent meta-analysis, apneic oxygenation was associated with a higher peri-intubation oxygen saturation, decreased rates of hypoxemia, and increased first-pass intubation success during emergency intubation in ICU and in the emergency department [32]. These results have been confirmed in another meta-analysis performed by Tan et al. in which apneic oxygenation with HFNC was associated with a decreased incidence of oxygen desaturation in emergency intubations [33]. It is clear that new studies are needed to clarify the efficacy of HFNC as a preoxygenation and oxygenation tool, and above all to identify the category of patients that can benefit the most. Based on these findings, 2019 guidelines of the French Society of Anesthesia and Intensive Care Medicine (SFAR) state that it is possible to use HFNC for preoxygenation in ICU, especially for patients not severely hypoxemic [34]. In a recent guideline, meta-analysis of ten trials performed both in the OR and the ICU showed that, when compared to COT and NIV, HFNC had no effect on the incidence of peri-intubation hypoxemia (i.e., $SpO_2 < 80\%$), 28-day mortality, serious complications, or ICU length of stay [35]. In addition, HFNC use had no effect on apneic time, PaO_2 measured both after preoxygenation and after intubation, or $PaCO_2$ measured after intubation when compared to COT or NIV. Finally, no recommendation was made regarding the use of HFNC in the peri-intubation period. For patients who are already receiving HFNC, the expert panel suggested continuing HFNC during intubation (conditional recommendation, moderate certainty) [35].

In conclusion, HFNC has been shown to be a promising tool for the prevention of oxygen desaturation in ICU patients, especially when combined with NIV (in the most severe) and when used in the less severely hypoxemic patients (Table 5.1). Other studies are needed to better clarify the impact of HFNC in specific patient populations, such as those with severe hypoxia, obesity, or difficult intubation and at high risk for desaturation.

5.3   Clinical Application of HFNC during Weaning from Mechanical Ventilation

5.3.1   Pathophysiology of Weaning Failure and Weaning Management

Liberating a patient from invasive mechanical ventilation is an important daily challenge in the ICU.

According to the new definition proposed by the WIND Study, successful weaning is represented by extubation without death or reintubation within 7 days (whether postextubation noninvasive ventilation was used or not), or ICU discharge without invasive mechanical ventilation within 7 days, whichever comes first [36]. Weaning failure may lead to reintubation resulting in increased mortality rates (25–50%), prolonged mechanical ventilation, increased incidence of ventilator-associated pneumonia, and longer ICU and hospital stays [12–16, 37]. Risk factors for weaning failure can be distinguished as [38]:

– *Factors related to patient and comorbidities*, such as age > 65 years [13, 39, 40], moderate or severe cardiorespiratory disease [13], and body-mass index >30 [41].
– *Factors related to acute pathology*, such as neurological disease [42], airway patency problem [40], inability to deal with respiratory secretions [40], APACHE II >12 on extubation day [14, 39], difficult or prolonged weaning [40], acute respiratory failure of cardiac origin [14], pneumonia as the reason for intubation [43], and positive fluid balance [43].
– *Factors related to functional parameters*, such as respiratory rate > 35 breaths/min [44], rapid shallow breathing index >105 [45], maximum inspiratory pressure (MIP) $\geq$ −20 to −25 cm H_2O [42, 44], peak expiratory flow <60 L/min [46], airway occlusion pressure at 0.1 s (P0.1) $\leq$4–5 cmH$_2$O [42], vital capacity (VC) $\leq$10 mL/kg [42, 44], and P0.1/MIP <0.3 [47].

Extubation and the subsequent passage from positive pressure mechanical ventilation to spontaneous breathing induce several pathophysiological changes that can lead to weaning failure, especially in high-risk patients. The main pathophysiological changes can be divided into changes in the airway status and changes in the cardiorespiratory status [38]. Upper airway obstruction is one of the common causes of extubation failure related to changes in airway status. It is frequently caused by laryngeal edema which can occur after extubation, resulting in a reduction of the airway diameter that leads to an increase of the resistive component of work of breathing, which may cause, consequently, respiratory distress [38, 48–50]. The quantitative cuff leak test is a screening test recommended before extubation in patients at risk of postextubation stridor [51]. If the test is considered positive (the difference between expiratory volume with inflated cuff and expiratory volume with deflated cuff less than 130 mL or the expiratory volume with deflated cuff less than 12% of the inspiratory volume), the administration of steroids, at least 4 h before extubation, might decrease laryngeal inflammation and edema [52]. Other less frequent causes of extubation failure related to impaired airway status are laryngospasm and excessive tracheobronchial secretions at the time of extubation associated to ineffective cough [38].

A loss of pulmonary aeration can occur during the passage from mechanical ventilation to spontaneous breathing. Atelectasis, alveolar transudation, and edema represent the main pathophysiological mechanisms associated with loss of lung aeration, which can lead to decreased lung compliance, ventilation-perfusion mismatch, and shunt effect [38, 53, 54]. Atelectasis is determined by the decrease in transpulmonary end-expiratory pressure which occurs during spontaneous breathing that can reduce lung volume to values below the closing capacity in unstable alveoli, thus determining their collapse [38]. The heterogeneity of the lung parenchyma due to atelectasis could lead to elevated regional driving transpulmonary pressure (i.e., the difference between end-inspiratory transpulmonary pressure and end-expiratory transpulmonary pressure), worsening of lung injury, pulmonary edema, and respiratory distress [53, 54]. Alveolar transudation and edema after extubation are caused by increased difference between intravascular capillary pressure and alveolar pressure and by increased cardiac output.

The discontinuation of positive mechanical ventilation can cause pronounced negative swings in intrathoracic pressure, depending on the patient's inspiratory effort, thus resulting in an increased left ventricular transmural pressure and afterload [38, 53–55]. Besides, the greater diaphragmatic excursion during spontaneous breathing associated to more negative values of intrathoracic pressure determines an increased transdiaphragmatic pressure (i.e., the difference between abdominal pressure and intrathoracic pressure) leading to increased venous return and right ventricular preload [38]. Consequently, this could determine a worsening of preexisting heart failure or its new onset. Furthermore, at the time of extubation, stimulation of airway receptors causes increased sympathetic activity, which might result in hypertension, increased heart rate, and arrhythmias [38, 56, 57].

Diaphragmatic weakness, injury, and atrophy occur rapidly during mechanical ventilation in critically ill patients [58]. Adequate neuromuscular function is another important factor for successful weaning [44]. Ventilatory assistance suppressing inspiratory effort results in rapid diaphragm atrophy; on the other hand, insufficient ventilatory support may fail to adequately unload the respiratory muscles, potentially resulting in load-induced diaphragmatic inflammation and injury [59]. As a result, an imbalance between the respiratory muscle's capacity and the respiratory load can occur during spontaneous breathing, with increased work of breathing and more CO_2 production, worsening of oxygenation, and clinical manifestations of respiratory distress such as use of accessory respiratory muscles, paradoxical breathing, and rapid shallow breathing. In addition, hypoxia and metabolic acidosis impair respiratory muscle function and cardiac function, triggering a vicious circle that, in the absence of adequate therapeutic measures, can lead to cardiorespiratory arrest [37, 38].

Early recognition of patients who are ready to begin the process of weaning from mechanical ventilation and identification of patients at higher risk of extubation failure allows implementation of strategies to prevent unsuccessful weaning.

Three strategies of ventilatory support can be used during the peri-extubation period [38, 60]:

- *Facilitative*, in selected patients who have failed the spontaneous breathing trial, to allow an early extubation with the aim of reducing the duration of invasive ventilation and its associated complications.
- *Preventive*, in selected and unselected patients, to prevent the onset of postextubation acute respiratory failure.
- *Therapeutic*, in patients with postextubation acute respiratory failure, to avoid reintubation.

These strategies are implemented using several ventilatory support techniques, such as COT, NIV, continuous positive airway pressure (CPAP), and HFNC, selecting the most appropriate ones according to the different patient categories [38, 61]. Patients are, in fact, distinguished as medical and surgical patients, on the basis of the ICU admission diagnosis, and also as high-risk and low-risk patients on the basis of risk factors for extubation failure (mainly age > 65 years, and underlying cardiac or respiratory disease) [38].

5.3.2 HFNC Clinical Application during Weaning Process in Surgical Patients

No studies are currently available regarding the application of HFNC as *facilitative strategy* during weaning process in surgical patients. Only a post hoc analysis of the Bilevel Positive Airway Pressure Versus Optiflow study (BiPOP study) suggested that facilitative HFNC or NIV had a similar effect on the likelihood of treatment failure in patients who underwent cardiothoracic surgery (28% for HFNC vs. 41% for NIV, respectively, $p = 0.33$), but too few patients were included for any meaningful conclusion on this issue [62, 63].

Several studies have reported the *preventive use* of HFNC during weaning process in surgical patients. Preventive strategies should be considered in case of a high risk of postextubation acute respiratory failure. Different techniques can be used selecting the most appropriate ones based on the type of surgery. The Bilevel Positive Airway Pressure Versus Optiflow study is a non-inferiority trial in which HFNC and NIV were compared in the postoperative setting of patients undergoing cardiothoracic surgery. NIV and HFNC were applied according to three different strategies: facilitative, preventive, or therapeutic. This trial showed that HFNC is not inferior to NIV, since treatment failure, defined as reintubation, switch to the other treatment, or premature discontinuation, was similar in both groups (21% for HFNC and 21.9% for NIV, for the three strategies combined; absolute risk difference 0.9%, 95% CI −4.9% to 6.6%, $p = 0.003$), as were reintubations (14% in both groups). Besides, when considered as preventive strategies, treatment failure was lower in the HFNC group (6%) than in the NIV group (13%; $p = 0.04$) [38, 62].

Few studies have compared HFNC and COT as preventive strategies in patients undergoing cardiac and thoracic surgery reporting conflicting results regarding the effect of HFNC on atelectasis and oxygenation [64–68]. Corley and coworkers have evaluated the preventive use of HFNC (gas flow rate of 50 L/min) as compared to COT in 20 patients after cardiac surgery [37, 64]. They found improved oxygenation and reduced respiratory rate and dyspnea in patients treated with HFNC. The same authors conducted a randomized, controlled trial in 155 obese patients (BMI ≥ 30) undergoing cardiac surgery to verify if preventive HFNC as compared to COT can reduce postoperative atelectasis assessed using Radiological Atelectasis Score on the chest X-ray [68]. Atelectasis rate, as well as secondary outcomes (oxygenation, respiratory rate, treatment failure, and ICU length of stay), was not different between the two groups, probably because chest X-ray is not accurate as compared to computed tomography to measure atelectasis and also because treatment time was too short (8 h) to highlight HFNC advantages [37, 68]. These results are in line with those of Parke and colleagues who have found no significant difference between preventive HFNC and COT in oxygenation, respiratory rate, cardiovascular parameters, atelectasis score, and hospital and ICU length of stay in patients undergoing cardiac surgery while a lower escalation in respiratory support due to acute respiratory failure was reported in the HFNC group (38% for HFNC vs. 62% for COT), although this study was not powered for this outcome [65].

After thoracic surgery, two studies showed a reduction in reintubation rate and hospital length of stay with HFNC use as compared to COT; however these studies were not powered for these outcomes [66, 67]. The potential usefulness of preventive HFNC in patients undergoing major abdominal surgery is unclear, as reported by the OPERA trial. In this study, HFNC and COT are compared in patients undergoing major abdominal surgery at medium-high risk of postoperative pulmonary complications [69]. No difference was found in the proportion of patients with hypoxemia ($PaO_2/FiO_2 \leq 300$) at 1 h after extubation and at treatment discontinuation, postoperative pulmonary complications, duration of hospital stay, and hospital mortality. Given the paucity of the available data, further studies are needed to assess the effect of preventive HFNC in this type of surgery.

The potential benefits of preventive HFNC compared to COT in surgical patients are unclear, regardless of the type of surgery. These conflicting results may be due to several factors, such as the shorter treatment duration in surgical patients, since, although the optimal treatment time has not been defined, it is known that the oxygenation improvement due to lung recruitment is more evident after at least 24 h of treatment. In addition, in the studies conducted on surgical patients, gas flow rate is lower than that set in medical patients probably because surgical patients do not have peak inspiratory flow as high as that found in medical patients, thus underestimating potential beneficial effect of HFNC [37].

In the postoperative setting, the use of HFNC as *therapeutic strategy* has been reported in patients developing ARF after cardiothoracic surgery [63]. A post hoc analysis of the Bilevel Positive Airway Pressure Versus Optiflow trial showed no differences in treatment failure between HFNC and NIV (27% for HFNC vs. 28% for NIV, $p = 0.93$) [63]. This might suggest that postoperative HFNC can be used as a first-line, noninvasive technique of respiratory support after cardiothoracic surgery because it is non-inferior to NIV [38]. No data are available for the therapeutic use of HFNC in other type of surgical patients.

A recent guideline analyzed the results of 11 trials performed in postoperative patients comparing HFNC versus COT (ten trials) or NIV (one trial) [35]. Compared to COT, postoperative HFNC use was associated with a significantly lower reintubation rate (relative risk [RR] 0.32 [0.12–0.88, moderate certainty]) and decreased need to escalate respiratory support (RR 0.54 [0.31–0.94, very low certainty]) while HFNC had no effect on mortality (low certainty), ICU length of stay (high certainty), hospital length of stay (moderate certainty), or incidence of postoperative hypoxia (low certainty). A post hoc subgroup analysis, comparing high-risk (combination of obese patients and those at high risk of postoperative respiratory complication) vs. non-high-risk patients, showed increased benefit of HFNC for high-risk patients. When compared to NIV, HFNC had no effect on the reintubation rate (low certainty), need for respiratory support (low certainty), or ICU length of stay (low certainty).

On the basis of these findings, the guideline suggested using HFNC compared to COT to prevent respiratory failure in the immediate postoperative period in high-risk and/or obese patients undergoing cardiac or thoracic surgery (conditional recommendation, moderate certainty evidence). The guidelines suggested, however, against prophylactic HFNC use to prevent respiratory failure in other postoperative patients (conditional recommendation, very low certainty evidence) [35] (Table 5.1).

5.3.3 HFNC Application during Weaning Process in Critically Ill Patients

No data are available regarding the *facilitative* use of HFNC in critically ill patients. NIV is the only respiratory support technique that can be used for facilitative purposes; several studies have shown its efficacy in patients with chronic obstructive pulmonary disease (COPD) or hypercapnia [38, 61, 70–76].

In low-risk medical patients, HFNC is the preferable *preventive* strategy if the device is available, given the advantages over COT as shown in several studies [38, 41, 77, 78]. Maggiore et al. have conducted the first randomized controlled trial to compare the effect of Venturi mask and HFNC (gas flow rate of 50 L/min) in moderate hypoxemic patients (i.e., $PaO_2/FiO_2 \leq 300$ at the beginning of spontaneous breathing trial) for the first 48 h after extubation on the PaO_2/FiO_2 ratio, patient discomfort, and other clinical outcomes [77]. The authors found that for the same delivered FiO_2, HFNC group reported significantly higher PaO_2/FiO_2 at 24, 36, and 48 h, underlining that the improvement in the PaO_2/FiO_2 ratio is a time-dependent phenomenon linked to HFNC efficacy on atelectasis [77]. Decreased $PaCO_2$, statistically significant at 3 h after extubation (32 mmHg vs. 36 mmHg), and lower respiratory rate (mean difference of 4 ± 1 breaths/min) were found in the HFNC group, probably related to the reduction in the upper airways dead space and in the work of breathing [77]. In addition, as compared to Venturi mask group, patients treated with HFNC experienced less discomfort, fewer displacements of the interface, fewer desaturations, and also fewer rate of postextubation acute respiratory failure requiring any form of ventilator support (8% vs. 35%), with less need for NIV (4% vs. 15%) and endotracheal reintubation (4% vs. 21%).

Hernàndez and coworkers did a multicenter randomized controlled trial enrolling 527 mechanically ventilated patients (medical and surgical) at low risk for extubation failure to assess the effects of HFNC (average flow rate of 31 L/min) and COT (delivered through nasal cannula or non-rebreathing face mask) applied for 24 h after extubation to prevent reintubation [41]. They found that HFNC use was associated with a reduced reintubation rate at 72 h (5% vs. 12%, $p = 0.004$), lower postextubation acute respiratory failure (8% vs. 14%, $p = 0.03$), and decreased laryngeal edemas requiring intubation (0% vs. 3%, $p = 0.001$), while time to reintubation was similar in both groups [41]. The two aforementioned studies were included in a recent meta-analysis which showed that HFNC significantly decreased the reintubation frequency compared with COT (RR 0.35, 95% CI 0.19–0.64; $p = 0.0007$), representing an attractive approach to prevent postextubation acute respiratory failure in unselected ICU patients [38, 78].

In 604 medical patients at high risk for postextubation respiratory failure, Hernàndez et al. conducted a non-inferiority randomized controlled trial to compare the preventive use of HFNC and NIV applied for 24 h after extubation to avert the risk of postextubation acute respiratory failure [79]. HFNC was not inferior to NIV in preventing reintubation (22.8 vs. 19.1%; absolute risk difference − 3.7; 95% CI −9.1 to ∞; in the multivariable analysis, the marginal odds ratio was 1.25; 95% CI 0–1.74). The postextubation acute respiratory failure at 72 h was higher in the NIV group (39.8% for NIV vs. 26.9% for HFNC; absolute risk difference 12.9; 95% CI 6.6 to ∞), probably because of greater patient discomfort which resulted in a lower treatment compliance. This seems also confirmed by a shorter than planned treatment duration in the NIV group as compared to HFNC (14 h, instead of 24 h as intended in the study protocol) [79]. Therefore, HFNC can be an effective alternative to NIV for preventing acute respiratory failure in high-risk patients, although further investigation is needed. In another randomized, controlled trial, Thille and coworkers compared the effects of HFNC alone or HFNC with NIV immediately after extubation in 641 patients at high risk of extubation failure (i.e., older than 65 years or with an underlying cardiac or respiratory disease) [80]. They found that the reintubation rate at day 7 was significantly reduced with HFNC and NIV, as compared to HFNC alone (11.8% vs. 18.2%, difference − 6.4% [95% CI, −12.0% to −0.9%], $p = 0.02$), as well as the postextubation respiratory failure rate at day 7 (21% vs. 29%; difference − 8.7% [95% CI, −15.2% to −1.8%], $p = 0.01$), thus suggesting that the combination of HFNC and NIV can be particularly useful in high-risk patients.

One study has compared HFNC (gas flow rate of 40 L/min) and COT (through nasal prongs or Venturi mask) to prevent postextubation acute respiratory failure in high-risk non-hypercapnic patients. The authors found that HFNC might be independently associated with lower postextubation failure after adjustment for confounding variables in four multivariable regression models. However this study is inconclusive because it is stopped for lower-than-planned patient enrollment [81].

Currently, no studies are available regarding the use of HFNC as a *therapeutic* strategy in critically ill patients.

A recent guideline analyzed the results of eight trials comparing the use of HFNC versus COT (five trials) or NIV (three trials) after extubation [35]. Compared to COT, HFNC reduced reintubation (RR 0.46 [0.30–0.70, moderate certainty]) and reduced postextubation respiratory failure (RR 0.52 [0.30–0.91, very low certainty]). Compared to NIPPV, HFNC had no effect on the rates of reintubation (low certainty) or postextubation respiratory failure (very low certainty). There were no effects of HFNC vs. COT or NIV on mortality (moderate certainty), need for escalation to NIV (moderate certainty, COT comparison only), or ICU (moderate certainty) and hospital LOS (moderate certainty). Based on these findings, the guideline suggested using HFNC compared to COT to prevent respiratory failure following extubation for patients who are intubated for more than 24 h and have any high-risk feature (conditional recommendation, moderate certainty evidence). For patients who clinicians would normally extubate to NIPPV, the experts' panel suggested continued use of NIPPV as opposed to HFNC (conditional recommendation, low certainty evidence) [35] (Table 5.1).

As for any postextubation respiratory support techniques, the use of HFNC after extubation should not delay intubation and escalation to invasive mechanical ventilation when this is more appropriate, because intubation delay can worsen the patient outcome and increase mortality [38].

Use of clinical scores can be helpful to predict HFNC outcome. Particularly, the ROX index (Respiratory rate-OXygenation), defined as the ratio of SpO_2/FiO_2 (which has a positive association with HFNC success) to respiratory rate (which has an inverse association), is validated to predict the outcome of HFNC therapy in critically ill patients with acute respiratory failure due to pneumonia [82]. A ROX index value measured at 12 h of treatment ≥ 4.88 identifies patients with a high chance of success while a value <3.85 is indicative for a high risk of failure and, therefore, intubation should be considered [82]. In addition, the dynamic of changes of its value may help discriminating those patients who will succeed with HFNC from those patients who will fail [82]. HFNC set flow rate significantly impacts oxygenation and respiratory rate in patients with acute respiratory failure [83]. On this basis, Mauri and colleagues conducted a physiological study to assess if the ROX index can be acutely modified by increasing the set flow rate during HFNC [84]. The authors found that more severe patients, characterized by lower SatO2/FiO2, higher respiratory rate, and lower ROX index at 30 L/min, showed larger benefits by increasing HFNC flow rate. The change of ROX index during a 20-min "flow challenge" might be helpful to identify more severe patients, likely needing closer monitoring [84].

5.4   Conclusion

Endotracheal intubation and mechanical ventilation represent a fundamental practice in anesthesia and critical care. HFNC is a powerful tool that has the potential to improve patient safety and clinical outcomes both in the preoxygenation phase of standard and emergency intubation and during the process of weaning from mechanical ventilation (Table 5.1).

HFNC can prevent adverse events related to intubation and may be used in surgical patients for providing apneic oxygenation during laryngoscopy and endotracheal tube positioning, especially in high-risk patients. Critical care patients might also benefit from HFNC during intubation, particularly the less severely hypoxemic patients.

Weaning failure may worsen patient's outcome and HFNC can be useful also in this context. In the postoperative setting, the HFNC use to prevent postextubation failure can be advised in high-risk and in obese patients undergoing cardiac or thoracic surgery. In the intensive care setting, weaning failure can be common in high-risk patients. Studies have demonstrated that HFNC, as compared to COT, can improve oxygenation, decrease the rate of postextubation respiratory failure, and reduce endotracheal intubation. When combined with NIV, HFNC can also decrease the reintubation rate in patients at higher risk for postextubation respiratory failure.

References

1. Weingart SD, Levitan RM. Preoxygenation and prevention of desaturation during emergency airway management. Ann Emerg Med. 2012;59(3):165–75. e1
2. Vourc'h M, Huard D, Feuillet F, Baud G, Guichoux A, Surbled M, et al. Preoxygenation in difficult airway management: high-flow oxygenation by nasal cannula versus face mask (the PREOPTIDAM study). Protocol for a single-Centre randomised study. BMJ Open. 2019;9(4):e025909.
3. Frerk C, Mitchell VS, McNarry AF, Mendonca C, Bhagrath R, Patel A, et al. Difficult Airway Society 2015 guidelines for management of unanticipated difficult intubation in adults. Br J Anaesth. 2015;115(6):827–48.
4. Guitton C, Ehrmann S, Volteau C, Colin G, Maamar A, Jean-Michel V, et al. Nasal high-flow preoxygenation for endotracheal intubation in the critically ill patient: a randomized clinical trial. Intensive Care Med. 2019;45(4):447–58.
5. Nimmagadda U, Salem MR, Crystal GJ. Preoxygenation: physiologic basis, benefits, and potential risks. Anesth Analg. 2017;124(2):507–17.
6. Baillard C, Fosse JP, Sebbane M, Chanques G, Vincent F, Courouble P, et al. Noninvasive ventilation improves preoxygenation before intubation of hypoxic patients. Am J Respir Crit Care Med. 2006;174(2):171–7.
7. Jaber S, Monnin M, Girard M, Conseil M, Cisse M, Carr J, et al. Apnoeic oxygenation via high-flow nasal cannula oxygen combined with non-invasive ventilation preoxygenation for intubation in hypoxaemic patients in the intensive care unit: the single-centre, blinded, randomised controlled OPTINIV trial. Intensive Care Med. 2016;42(12):1877–87.
8. Gleason JM, Christian BR, Barton ED. Nasal cannula apneic oxygenation prevents desaturation during endotracheal intubation: an integrative literature review. West J Emerg Med. 2018;19(2):403–11.

9. Miguel-Montanes R, Hajage D, Messika J, Bertrand F, Gaudry S, Rafat C, et al. Use of high-flow nasal cannula oxygen therapy to prevent desaturation during tracheal intubation of intensive care patients with mild-to-moderate hypoxemia. Crit Care Med. 2015;43(3):574–83.

10. Sakles JC, Mosier JM, Patanwala AE, Dicken JM. Apneic oxygenation is associated with a reduction in the incidence of hypoxemia during the RSI of patients with intracranial hemorrhage in the emergency department. Intern Emerg Med. 2016;11(7):983–92.

11. Papazian L, Corley A, Hess D, Fraser JF, Frat JP, Guitton C, et al. Use of high-flow nasal cannula oxygenation in ICU adults: a narrative review. Intensive Care Med. 2016;42(9):1336–49.

12. Thille AW, Richard JC, Brochard L. The decision to extubate in the intensive care unit. Am J Respir Crit Care Med. 2013;187(12):1294–302.

13. Thille AW, Harrois A, Schortgen F, Brun-Buisson C, Brochard L. Outcomes of extubation failure in medical intensive care unit patients. Crit Care Med. 2011;39(12):2612–8.

14. Epstein SK, Ciubotaru RL, Wong JB. Effect of failed extubation on the outcome of mechanical ventilation. Chest. 1997;112(1):186–92.

15. Esteban A, Alia I, Gordo F, Fernandez R, Solsona JF, Vallverdu I, et al. Extubation outcome after spontaneous breathing trials with T-tube or pressure support ventilation. The Spanish Lung Failure Collaborative Group. Am J Respir Crit Care Med. 1997;156(2 Pt 1):459–65.

16. Frutos-Vivar F, Esteban A, Apezteguia C, Gonzalez M, Arabi Y, Restrepo MI, et al. Outcome of reintubated patients after scheduled extubation. J Crit Care. 2011;26(5):502–9.

17. Patel A, Nouraei SA. Transnasal humidified rapid-insufflation Ventilatory exchange (THRIVE): a physiological method of increasing apnoea time in patients with difficult airways. Anaesthesia. 2015;70(3):323–9.

18. Booth AWG, Vidhani K, Lee PK, Thomsett CM. SponTaneous respiration using IntraVEnous anaesthesia and Hi-flow nasal oxygen (STRIVE Hi) maintains oxygenation and airway patency during management of the obstructed airway: an observational study. Br J Anaesth. 2017;118(3):444–51.

19. Doyle AJ, Stolady D, Mariyaselvam M, Wijewardena G, Gent E, Blunt M, et al. Preoxygenation and apneic oxygenation using transnasal humidified rapid-insufflation ventilatory exchange for emergency intubation. J Crit Care. 2016;36:8–12.

20. Badiger S, John M, Fearnley RA, Ahmad I. Optimizing oxygenation and intubation conditions during awake fibre-optic intubation using a high-flow nasal oxygen-delivery system. Br J Anaesth. 2015;115(4):629–32.

21. Raineri SM, Cortegiani A, Accurso G, Procaccianti C, Vitale F, Caruso S, et al. Efficacy and safety of using high-flow nasal oxygenation in patients undergoing rapid sequence intubation. Turkish J Anaesthesiol Reanim. 2017;45(6):335–9.

22. Heinrich SHT, Stubner B, et al. Benefits of heated and humidified high flow nasal oxygen for preoxygenation in morbidly obese patients undergoing bariatric surgery: a randomised controlled study. J Obes Bariatrics. 2014;I(I):7–13.

23. Vukovic AA, Hanson HR, Murphy SL, Mercurio D, Sheedy CA, Arnold DH. Apneic oxygenation reduces hypoxemia during endotracheal intubation in the pediatric emergency department. Am J Emerg Med. 2019;37(1):27–32.

24. Moller W, Feng S, Domanski U, Franke KJ, Celik G, Bartenstein P, et al. Nasal high flow reduces dead space. J Appl Physiol (1985). 2017;122(1):191–7.

25. Vourc'h M, Asfar P, Volteau C, Bachoumas K, Clavieras N, Egreteau PY, et al. High-flow nasal cannula oxygen during endotracheal intubation in hypoxemic patients: a randomized controlled clinical trial. Intensive Care Med. 2015;41(9):1538–48.

26. Semler MW, Janz DR, Lentz RJ, Matthews DT, Norman BC, Assad TR, et al. Randomized trial of apneic oxygenation during endotracheal intubation of the critically ill. Am J Respir Crit Care Med. 2016;193(3):273–80.

27. Ng I, Krieser R, Mezzavia P, Lee K, Tseng C, Douglas N, et al. The use of transnasal humidified rapid-insufflation ventilatory exchange (THRIVE) for pre-oxygenation in neurosurgical patients: a randomised controlled trial. Anaesth Intensive Care. 2018;46(4):360–7.

28. Tan PCF, Millay OJ, Leeton L, Dennis AT. High-flow humidified nasal preoxygenation in pregnant women: a prospective observational study. Br J Anaesth. 2019;122(1):86–91.

29. Renda T, Corrado A, Iskandar G, Pelaia G, Abdalla K, Navalesi P. High-flow nasal oxygen therapy in intensive care and anaesthesia. Br J Anaesth. 2018;120(1):18–27.

30. Mauri T, Wang YM, Dalla Corte F, Corcione N, Spinelli E, Pesenti A. Nasal high flow: physiology, efficacy and safety in the acute care setting, a narrative review. Open Access Emerg Med. 2019;11:109–20.

31. Frat JP, Ricard JD, Quenot JP, Pichon N, Demoule A, Forel JM, et al. Non-invasive ventilation versus high-flow nasal cannula oxygen therapy with apnoeic oxygenation for preoxygenation before intubation of patients with acute hypoxaemic respiratory failure: a randomised, multicentre, open-label trial. Lancet Respir Med. 2019;7(4):303–12.

32. Oliveira JESL, Cabrera D, Barrionuevo P, Johnson RL, Erwin PJ, Murad MH, et al. Effectiveness of apneic oxygenation during intubation: a systematic review and meta-analysis. Ann Emerg Med. 2017;70(4):483–94. e11

33. Tan E, Loubani O, Kureshi N, Green RS. Does apneic oxygenation prevent desaturation during emergency airway management? A systematic review and meta-analysis. Canadian J Anaesth. 2018;65(8):936–49.

34. Quintard H, l'Her E, Pottecher J, Adnet F, Constantin JM, De Jong A, et al. Experts' guidelines of intubation and extubation of the ICU patient of French Society of Anaesthesia and Intensive Care Medicine (SFAR) and French-speaking Intensive Care Society (SRLF): In collaboration with the pediatric Association of French-speaking Anaesthetists and Intensivists (ADARPEF), French-speaking Group of Intensive Care and Paediatric emergencies (GFRUP) and Intensive Care physiotherapy society (SKR). Ann Intensive Care. 2019;9(1):13.

35. Rochwerg B, Einav S, Chaudhuri D, Mancebo J, Mauri T, Helviz Y, et al. The role for high flow nasal cannula as a respiratory support strategy in adults: a clinical practice guideline. Intensive Care Med. 2020;46(12):2226–37.

36. Beduneau G, Pham T, Schortgen F, Piquilloud L, Zogheib E, Jonas M, et al. Epidemiology of weaning outcome according to a new definition. The WIND Study. Am J Respir Crit Care Med. 2017;195(6):772–83.

37. Braunlich. basics and modern practice of nasal high-flow therapy. First ed: UNI-MED; 2019.

38. Maggiore SM, Battilana M, Serano L, Petrini F. Ventilatory support after extubation in critically ill patients. Lancet Respir Med. 2018;6(12):948–62.

39. Ferrer M, Valencia M, Nicolas JM, Bernadich O, Badia JR, Torres A. Early noninvasive ventilation averts extubation failure in patients at risk: a randomized trial. Am J Respir Crit Care Med. 2006;173(2):164–70.

40. Nava S, Gregoretti C, Fanfulla F, Squadrone E, Grassi M, Carlucci A, et al. Noninvasive ventilation to prevent respiratory failure after extubation in high-risk patients. Crit Care Med. 2005;33(11):2465–70.

41. Hernandez G, Vaquero C, Gonzalez P, Subira C, Frutos-Vivar F, Rialp G, et al. Effect of postextubation high-flow nasal cannula vs conventional oxygen therapy on reintubation in low-risk patients: a randomized clinical trial. JAMA. 2016;315(13):1354–61.

42. Vallverdu I, Calaf N, Subirana M, Net A, Benito S, Mancebo J. Clinical characteristics, respiratory functional parameters, and outcome of a two-hour T-piece trial in patients weaning from mechanical ventilation. Am J Respir Crit Care Med. 1998;158(6):1855–62.

43. Frutos-Vivar F, Ferguson ND, Esteban A, Epstein SK, Arabi Y, Apezteguia C, et al. Risk factors for extubation failure in patients following a successful spontaneous breathing trial. Chest. 2006;130(6):1664–71.

44. Boles JM, Bion J, Connors A, Herridge M, Marsh B, Melot C, et al. Weaning from mechanical ventilation. Eur Respir J. 2007;29(5):1033–56.

45. Yang KL, Tobin MJ. A prospective study of indexes predicting the outcome of trials of weaning from mechanical ventilation. N Engl J Med. 1991;324(21):1445–50.

46. Smina M, Salam A, Khamiees M, Gada P, Amoateng-Adjepong Y, Manthous CA. Cough peak flows and extubation outcomes. Chest. 2003;124(1):262–8.

47. Capdevila XJ, Perrigault PF, Perey PJ, Roustan JP, d'Athis F. Occlusion pressure and its ratio to maximum inspiratory pressure are useful predictors for successful extubation following T-piece weaning trial. Chest. 1995;108(2):482–9.

48. Jaber S, Chanques G, Matecki S, Ramonatxo M, Vergne C, Souche B, et al. Post-extubation stridor in intensive care unit patients. Risk factors evaluation and importance of the cuff-leak test. Intensive Care Med. 2003;29(1):69–74.
49. Straus C, Louis B, Isabey D, Lemaire F, Harf A, Brochard L. Contribution of the endotracheal tube and the upper airway to breathing workload. Am J Respir Crit Care Med. 1998;157(1):23–30.
50. Pluijms WA, van Mook WN, Wittekamp BH, Bergmans DC. Postextubation laryngeal edema and stridor resulting in respiratory failure in critically ill adult patients: updated review. Crit Care. 2015;19:295.
51. Girard TD, Alhazzani W, Kress JP, Ouellette DR, Schmidt GA, Truwit JD, et al. An Official American Thoracic Society/American College of Chest Physicians Clinical Practice Guideline: liberation from mechanical ventilation in critically ill adults. Rehabilitation protocols, ventilator liberation protocols, and cuff leak tests. Am J Respir Crit Care Med. 2017;195(1):120–33.
52. Schmidt GA, Girard TD, Kress JP, Morris PE, Ouellette DR, Alhazzani W, et al. Official Executive Summary of an American Thoracic Society/American College of Chest Physicians Clinical Practice Guideline: liberation from mechanical ventilation in critically ill adults. Am J Respir Crit Care Med. 2017;195(1):115–9.
53. Mauri T, Grasselli G, Jaber S. Respiratory support after extubation: noninvasive ventilation or high-flow nasal cannula, as appropriate. Ann Intensive Care. 2017;7(1):52.
54. Soummer A, Perbet S, Brisson H, Arbelot C, Constantin JM, Lu Q, et al. Ultrasound assessment of lung aeration loss during a successful weaning trial predicts postextubation distress*. Crit Care Med. 2012;40(7):2064–72.
55. Navalesi P, Maggiore SM. Positive end-expiratory pressure. In: Tobin MJ, editor. Principles and practice of mechanical ventilation. 3rd ed. New York: McGraw-Hill, Inc.; 2012. p. 253–302.
56. Hamaya Y, Dohi S. Differences in cardiovascular response to airway stimulation at different sites and blockade of the responses by lidocaine. Anesthesiology. 2000;93(1):95–103.
57. Sharma VB, Prabhakar H, Rath GP, Bithal PK. Comparison of dexmedetomidine and lignocaine on attenuation of airway and pressor responses during tracheal extubation. J Neuroanaesthesiol Crit Care. 2014;1:50–5.
58. Jaber S, Petrof BJ, Jung B, Chanques G, Berthet JP, Rabuel C, et al. Rapidly progressive diaphragmatic weakness and injury during mechanical ventilation in humans. Am J Respir Crit Care Med. 2011;183(3):364–71.
59. Goligher EC, Dres M, Fan E, Rubenfeld GD, Scales DC, Herridge MS, et al. Mechanical ventilation-induced diaphragm atrophy strongly impacts clinical outcomes. Am J Respir Crit Care Med. 2018;197(2):204–13.
60. Antonelli M, Bello G. Noninvasive mechanical ventilation during the weaning process: facilitative, curative, or preventive? Crit Care. 2008;12(2):136.
61. Rochwerg B, Brochard L, Elliott MW, Hess D, Hill NS, Nava S, et al. Official ERS/ATS clinical practice guidelines: noninvasive ventilation for acute respiratory failure. Eur Respir J. 2017;50:2.
62. Stephan F, Barrucand B, Petit P, Rezaiguia-Delclaux S, Medard A, Delannoy B, et al. High-flow nasal oxygen vs. noninvasive positive airway pressure in hypoxemic patients after cardiothoracic surgery: a randomized clinical trial. JAMA. 2015;313(23):2331–9.
63. Stephan F. High-flow nasal oxygen therapy for postextubation acute hypoxemic respiratory failure—reply. JAMA. 2015;314(15):1644–5.
64. Corley A, Caruana LR, Barnett AG, Tronstad O, Fraser JF. Oxygen delivery through high-flow nasal cannulae increase end-expiratory lung volume and reduce respiratory rate in post-cardiac surgical patients. Br J Anaesth. 2011;107(6):998–1004.
65. Parke R, McGuinness S, Dixon R, Jull A. Open-label, phase II study of routine high-flow nasal oxygen therapy in cardiac surgical patients. Br J Anaesth. 2013;111(6):925–31.
66. Yu Y, Qian X, Liu C, Zhu C. Effect of high-flow nasal cannula versus conventional oxygen therapy for patients with thoracoscopic lobectomy after extubation. Can Respir J. 2017;2017:7894631.

67. Ansari BM, Hogan MP, Collier TJ, Baddeley RA, Scarci M, Coonar AS, et al. A randomized controlled trial of high-flow nasal oxygen (Optiflow) as part of an enhanced recovery program after lung resection surgery. Ann Thorac Surg. 2016;101(2):459–64.

68. Corley A, Bull T, Spooner AJ, Barnett AG, Fraser JF. Direct extubation onto high-flow nasal cannulae post-cardiac surgery versus standard treatment in patients with a BMI >/=30: a randomised controlled trial. Intensive Care Med. 2015;41(5):887–94.

69. Futier E, Paugam-Burtz C, Godet T, Khoy-Ear L, Rozencwajg S, Delay JM, et al. Effect of early postextubation high-flow nasal cannula vs conventional oxygen therapy on hypoxaemia in patients after major abdominal surgery: a French multicentre randomised controlled trial (OPERA). Intensive Care Med. 2016;42(12):1888–98.

70. Nava S, Ambrosino N, Clini E, Prato M, Orlando G, Vitacca M, et al. Noninvasive mechanical ventilation in the weaning of patients with respiratory failure due to chronic obstructive pulmonary disease. A randomized, controlled trial. Ann Intern Med. 1998;128(9):721–8.

71. Vitacca M, Ambrosino N, Clini E, Porta R, Rampulla C, Lanini B, et al. Physiological response to pressure support ventilation delivered before and after extubation in patients not capable of totally spontaneous autonomous breathing. Am J Respir Crit Care Med. 2001;164(4):638–41.

72. Girault C, Daudenthun I, Chevron V, Tamion F, Leroy J, Bonmarchand G. Noninvasive ventilation as a systematic extubation and weaning technique in acute-on-chronic respiratory failure: a prospective, randomized controlled study. Am J Respir Crit Care Med. 1999;160(1):86–92.

73. Girault C, Bubenheim M, Abroug F, Diehl JL, Elatrous S, Beuret P, et al. Noninvasive ventilation and weaning in patients with chronic hypercapnic respiratory failure: a randomized multicenter trial. Am J Respir Crit Care Med. 2011;184(6):672–9.

74. Burns KE, Meade MO, Premji A, Adhikari NK. Noninvasive positive-pressure ventilation as a weaning strategy for intubated adults with respiratory failure. Cochrane Database Syst Rev. 2013;12:CD004127.

75. Burns KE, Meade MO, Premji A, Adhikari NK. Noninvasive ventilation as a weaning strategy for mechanical ventilation in adults with respiratory failure: a Cochrane systematic review. CMAJ. 2014;186(3):E112–22.

76. Ferrer M, Esquinas A, Arancibia F, Bauer TT, Gonzalez G, Carrillo A, et al. Noninvasive ventilation during persistent weaning failure: a randomized controlled trial. Am J Respir Crit Care Med. 2003;168(1):70–6.

77. Maggiore SM, Idone FA, Vaschetto R, Festa R, Cataldo A, Antonicelli F, et al. Nasal high-flow versus Venturi mask oxygen therapy after extubation. Effects on oxygenation, comfort, and clinical outcome. Am J Respir Crit Care Med. 2014;190(3):282–8.

78. Huang HW, Sun XM, Shi ZH, Chen GQ, Chen L, Friedrich JO, et al. Effect of high-flow nasal cannula oxygen therapy versus conventional oxygen therapy and noninvasive ventilation on reintubation rate in adult patients after extubation: a systematic review and meta-analysis of randomized controlled trials. J Intensive Care Med. 2017; 885066617705118

79. Hernandez G, Vaquero C, Colinas L, Cuena R, Gonzalez P, Canabal A, et al. Effect of postextubation high-flow nasal cannula vs noninvasive ventilation on reintubation and postextubation respiratory failure in high-risk patients: a randomized clinical trial. JAMA. 2016;316(15):1565–74.

80. Thille AW, Muller G, Gacouin A, Coudroy R, Decavele M, Sonneville R, et al. Effect of postextubation high-flow nasal oxygen with noninvasive ventilation vs high-flow nasal oxygen alone on reintubation among patients at high risk of Extubation failure: a randomized clinical trial. JAMA. 2019;322(15):1465–75.

81. Fernandez R, Subira C, Frutos-Vivar F, Rialp G, Laborda C, Masclans JR, et al. High-flow nasal cannula to prevent postextubation respiratory failure in high-risk non-hypercapnic patients: a randomized multicenter trial. Ann Intensive Care. 2017;7(1):47.

82. Roca O, Caralt B, Messika J, Samper M, Sztrymf B, Hernandez G, et al. An index combining respiratory rate and oxygenation to predict outcome of nasal high-flow therapy. Am J Respir Crit Care Med. 2019;199(11):1368–76.

83. Mauri T, Alban L, Turrini C, Cambiaghi B, Carlesso E, Taccone P, et al. Optimum support by high-flow nasal cannula in acute hypoxemic respiratory failure: effects of increasing flow rates. Intensive Care Med. 2017;43(10):1453–63.
84. Mauri T, Carlesso E, Spinelli E, Turrini C, Corte FD, Russo R, et al. Increasing support by nasal high flow acutely modifies the ROX index in hypoxemic patients: a physiologic study. J Crit Care. 2019;53:183–5.

Clinical Applications of High-Flow Nasal Cannula in the Operating Room

6

Audrey De Jong, Amélie Rollé, Laurie Ducros, Yassir Aarab, Clément Monet, and Samir Jaber

In operative rooms, high-flow nasal cannula oxygen (HFNO) can be used in various settings: during the intubation procedure (for preoxygenation and/or apneic oxygenation) or during procedures without intubation (oropharyngeal surgeries, digestive upper or lower endoscopy). When used in operating rooms, HFNO is often called "transnasal humidified rapid-insufflation ventilatory exchange (THRIVE)." The potential indications for using HFNO (THRIVE) in operating room are summarized in Fig. 6.1.

A. De Jong
PhyMedExp, University of Montpellier, INSERM U1046, CNRS UMR 9214, Montpellier, France

Anesthesia and Critical Care Department B, Saint Eloi Teaching Hospital, Centre Hospitalier Universitaire Montpellier, Montpellier cedex 5, France

A. Rollé · L. Ducros · Y. Aarab · C. Monet
Anesthesia and Critical Care Department B, Saint Eloi Teaching Hospital, Centre Hospitalier Universitaire Montpellier, Montpellier cedex 5, France

S. Jaber (✉)
PhyMedExp, University of Montpellier, INSERM U1046, CNRS UMR 9214, Montpellier, France

Anesthesia and Critical Care Department B, Saint Eloi Teaching Hospital, Centre Hospitalier Universitaire Montpellier, Montpellier cedex 5, France

Intensive Care Unit, Anaesthesia and Critical Care Department, Saint Eloi Teaching Hospital, University Montpellier 1, Montpellier, Cedex 5, France
e-mail: s-jaber@chu-montpellier.fr

© Springer Nature Switzerland AG 2021
A. Carlucci, S. M. Maggiore (eds.), *High Flow Nasal Cannula*,
https://doi.org/10.1007/978-3-030-42454-1_6

Fig. 6.1 Potential
indications for using
HFNO (THRIVE) in the
operating room

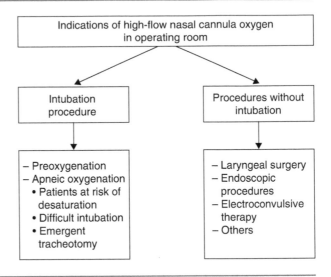

Fig. 6.1 Potential indications for using HFNO (THRIVE) in the operating room

6.1 During Intubation Procedure

Several preoxygenation maneuvers in spontaneous ventilation (3–8 vital capacities or 3 min of tidal volume ventilation) exist and seem to be of comparable effectiveness [1]. Some technical details, however, may be responsible for significant differences. First, the clinician must ensure that the mask is appropriate for the patient's morphology. Second, the fresh gas flow rate must be strong enough to homogenize pulmonary ventilation and reduce the impact of leaks. Thirdly, leaks must be avoided and diagnosed either in the case of an empty tank or by the absence of a normal capnography curve, as leaks alter the effectiveness of preoxygenation.

The expired oxygen concentration (EtO2) is used to evaluate the alveolar oxygen pressure (PaO_2). During preoxygenation, the commonly adopted objective of expired oxygen concentration is 90% [1, 2]. This objective is achieved more quickly when pure oxygen is administered. Although the clinician should be aware of the potential complications of denitrogenation, such as atelectasis, the benefit of maximum preoxygenation (oxygen-inspired fraction (FiO_2) = 100%) is greater than the risk of developing atelectasis.

HFNO, which provides a high flow rate, heated and moistened air through a nasal cannula to a 100% FiO_2, and a maximum flow rate of 60 L/min, can allow the passage of orotracheal tube through the mouth. Apneic oxygenation is a physiological phenomenon in which the difference between the alveolar rates of oxygen removal and carbon dioxide excretion generates a negative pressure gradient of up to 20 cmH2O. This negative pressure gradient allows the entry of oxygen into the lungs, provided that there is airway permeability between the lungs and the atmosphere. Clinical studies have evaluated the effect of apneic oxygenation, with conflicting results [3]. The apparent contradictory results of these studies [4–6] can be explained in part by differences in study types, oxygen therapy parameters, and patients included: the effectiveness of apneic oxygenation depends on the FiO_2 delivered, flow rate of oxygen, alveolar-capillary membrane, and degree of hypoxemia. The use of HFNO combined with noninvasive ventilation (NIV) may thus have potential advantages over NIV alone for preoxygenation prior to intubation procedures in hypoxemic patients. The preoxygenation technique combining NIV and HFNO, combining the notions of prevention of alveolar derecruitment and apneic oxygenation, respectively, was recently evaluated [7]. The lowest saturation during the intubation process was significantly higher using the combination of NIV and HFNO (OPTINIV method), compared with the NIV alone [7].

A physiologic study [8] performed in healthy volunteers associated preoxygenation with a bag-valve mask and nasal cannula. The aim of the study was to assess the optimum nasal cannula flow rate for preoxygenation or whether the presence of nasal cannula alone creates a mask leak. Nasal cannula 0 L/min and nasal cannula 5 L/min recorded significantly lower EtO2 at all times compared with nasal cannula 15 L/min, nasal cannula 10 L/min, or bag-valve mask only.

In the operating room, apneic oxygenation is evaluated. A first study investigated the influence of nasal oxygen delivery on the duration of arterial oxygen saturation (SpO2) $\geq$95% in simulated difficult laryngoscopy in obese patients [9]. Nasal administration of O_2 was associated with significant increases in SpO_2 frequency and duration $\geq$95% and higher minimal SpO_2 in prolonged laryngoscopies in obese patients. These results were confirmed in a randomized controlled study comparing HFNO and face mask preoxygenation [10]. However, no bag-valve mask ventilation was performed after induction in the face mask group.

In another study [11], 33 morbidly obese patients undergoing laparoscopic bariatric surgery were randomized to receive one of the following preoxygenation strategies for 7 min: HFNO, continuous positive airway pressure (CPAP), or oxygen insufflation via a standard face mask [11]. In all three groups, PaO_2 values were significantly increased at 1 and 3 min following preoxygenation. Maximum oxygenation levels were reached after 3 min of preoxygenation, with no significant increase thereafter. The standard group had a median arterial oxygen partial pressure level of 337 mmHg (295 mmHg–390 mmHg), the PPC group of 353 mmHg (293 mmHg–419 mmHg), and the HFNO group of 380 mmHg (339 mmHg–443 mmHg). This study suggests, despite its limitations, that high-speed humidified nasal oxygen could provide rapid, safe, and easy-to-use preoxygenation in obese patients prior to general anesthesia.

A randomized controlled trial [12], including 20 patients in each group, compared THRIVE preoxygenation to face mask preoxygenation in patients undergoing emergency surgery. Arterial blood gases were sampled from an arterial catheter immediately after intubation, showing no difference in mean PaO_2, $PaCO_2$, or pH. However, the study was not powered to find a difference in complications related to intubation. In a similar emergency surgery setting, in patients also undergoing rapid sequence induction, a recent study [13] showed that on 80 adult patients less desaturation events were observed with THRIVE for rapid sequence induction compared with face mask preoxygenation.

Another randomized controlled trial [14] assessed the use of HFNO in both preoxygenation and apneic oxygenation in adults who were intubated following a non-rapid sequence induction. Fifty patients were randomized to receive preoxygenation via a standard face mask or the THRIVE device. After 5 min of preoxygenation, induction and muscle-relaxant agents were given. While waiting for complete paralysis, patients in the standard face mask group received bag-mask ventilation, whereas patients in the HFNO group received apneic oxygenation via the THRIVE device. Serial blood samples for arterial blood gas analysis were taken. No complications were observed in either group. HFNO produces a higher PaO_2 after preoxygenation and safe PaO_2 during intubation. However, the subsequent fall in PaO_2 and rise in $PaCO_2$ indicate that HFNO was not as effective as bag-valve mask in maintaining oxygenation and ventilation following neuromuscular blockade.

Another preliminary study [15] found similar results. Group C patients ($n = 10$) were preoxygenated with 100% oxygen using a face mask at a rate of 6 L/min for 3 min with CPAP of 15 cm of H_2O. In Group H, oxygen was administered using THRIVE at 30 L/min for 3 min. Apneic ventilation was given in Group C with 10 L/min oxygen with CPAP of 15 cm H_2O and in Group H with THRIVE at 60 L/min. Both groups tolerated apnea for 12 min without desaturation. PaO_2 in Group C was significantly higher than Group H from 3 min of apnea to 12 min. The $PaCO_2$ was significantly lower in Group C from 6 min. The pH was comparable in both groups except at 12 min with Group H having significantly lower pH.

For preoxygenation of pregnant women, a recent prospective study [16] assessed a 3-min HFNO protocol (30 L min^{-1} for 30 s, and then 50 L min^{-1} for 150 s) for preoxygenation. The EtO_2 was assessed for the first four breaths after simulated preoxygenation. It was found that the proportion with first expired breath EtO2 $\geq$ 90% was 60% [95% confidence interval (CI): 54–66%] and EtO2 $\geq$ 80% was 84% (95% CI: 80–88%). HFNO using this protocol was inadequate to preoxygenate term pregnant women.

A very nice physiologic study [17] provided some explanations to the apparent discrepant results observed in the literature. When used as a method of preoxygenation, HFNO provides lower EtO2 than bag-valve mask [17]. Therefore, it seems that this method cannot replace preoxygenation using bag-valve mask or HFNO. Similarly, it cannot replace bag-valve mask ventilation, which allows a better ventilation of the patient than administration of oxygen only. However, it could be an interesting adjunct for apneic oxygenation, after the end of preoxygenation. This method was tested with success in intensive care unit (ICU) [7]. Further studies are needed in the operating room (Fig. 6.2).

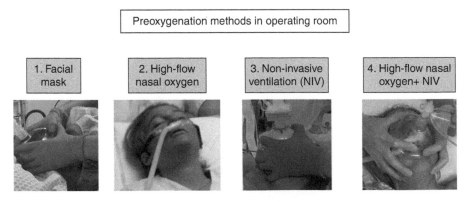

Fig. 6.2 Summarizes the different methods of preoxygenation available in the operating room

6.2   Procedures without Intubation

Another observational prospective study [18] assessed the apnea time of 25 patients with difficult planned intubation and undergoing general anesthesia for hypopharyngeal or laryngotracheal surgery. HFNO was administered continuously for preoxygenation and continued after intravenous induction of anesthesia and neuromuscular blockade, until airway safety was assured. The apnea time began during the administration of the neuromuscular blockers and ended with the beginning of the jet ventilation, positive pressure ventilation, or resumption of spontaneous ventilation. During this time, the permeability of the upper airway was ensured by dislocation of the jaw. Twenty-five patients were included, including 12 obese patients. The median apnea time was 14 (5–65) min. No arterial oxygen desaturation was observed during the apnea period.

In three patients who underwent laryngeal and tracheal surgeries under apneic conditions using transnasal humidified rapid-insufflation ventilatory exchange, transcutaneous CO_2 levels were recorded throughout the apneic period to detect the rates of CO_2 rise [19]. Conventional airway management was initiated after 15 minutes of apnea with either tracheal intubation or jet ventilation. No patient experienced oxygen desaturation <97%. The average rate of transcutaneous CO_2 rise (1.7 mm Hg/min) was higher than previously reported using this technique.

In a physiological study of apneic oxygenation using THRIVE during laryngeal surgery [20], it was shown that this technique is able to keep patients with mild systemic disease and a body mass index (BMI)<30 well oxygenated for a period of up to 30 min. Patients were well oxygenated, and SpO_2 was never below 91%. The increase in $PaCO_2$ and end-tidal CO_2 during apnea was 0.24 (0.05) and 0.12 (0.04) kPa min^{-1}, respectively. The THRIVE concept makes it possible to extend the apneic window but monitoring of CO_2 and/or pH is recommended.

In case of emergent awake surgical tracheostomy, because of a stridor for example, HFNO could also help to maintain oxygenation [21].

A promising area of application of HFNO is the management of general anesthesia during electroconvulsive therapy. Oxygenation is usually difficult after induction of the convulsions, and done using a simple face mask or low-flow nasal cannula. In a single-center feasibility study [22], 13 patients with a pharmacotherapy-resistant depressive disorder underwent 20 electroconvulsive therapy sessions with the use of THRIVE, without any desaturation.

Studies are ongoing about the interest of using HFNO rather than standard nasal cannula oxygen in endoscopy procedures, in particular digestive.

Nevertheless, the majority of studies were small, and their power was insufficient to detect respiratory events or other rare complications. Prolonged apnea oxygenation may be deleterious in patients with comorbidities such as increased intracranial pressure, metabolic acidosis, hyperkalemia, and pulmonary hypertension. Table 6.1 summarizes the advantages and inconvenience of THRIVE method during procedures without intubation.

Table 6.1 Advantages and inconvenience of using THRIVE in the operating room

Advantages	Inconvenience
Higher flow of humidified and warm oxygen compared to usual nasal cannula: May increase the safety of endoscopic procedures or electroconvulsive therapy	Discomfort associated with high flow
Apneic oxygenation during intubation procedure or other procedures	Increase of CO_2 during apnea period Major acidosis during apnea period Does not replace the bag-valve mask ventilation
Does not interfere with local surgery	Risk of fire in case of laser use
Avoid applying a facial mask for preoxygenation	Lower EtO2 than facial mask (preoxygenation)

EtO2 Expired fraction in oxygen, *CO_2* carbon dioxide

It is worth noting that a case of intraoral ignition of monopolar diathermy during THRIVE was reported [23]. This case highlights the need for maintained awareness of fire risk when using diathermy in the presence of THRIVE during airway surgery.

In a randomized controlled trial including 48 children [24], THRIVE exchange prolongs the safe apnea time in healthy children but has no effect to improve CO_2 clearance. In another randomized controlled trial including 60 children [25], the length of the safe apnea time using THRIVE with two different oxygen concentrations (100% vs. 30% oxygen) was not extended compared with standard low-flow 100% oxygen administration. Further studies are needed to confirm the safety and efficacy of THRIVE in children.

Acknowledgements Funding and Conflict of Interest: Support was provided solely from institutional and/or departmental sources.

Dr. Jaber reports receiving consulting fees from Drager, Xenios, and Fisher & Paykel. A. De Jong reports personal fees from Baxter and Medtronic, and travel reimbursements from Fresenius-Kabi, MSD France, Astellas, Pfizer, and Fisher & Paykel.

References

1. De Jong A, Futier E, Millot A, Coisel Y, Jung B, Chanques G, et al. How to preoxygenate in operative room: healthy subjects and situations "at risk". Ann Fr Anesth Reanim. 2014;33(7–8):457–61.
2. De Jong A, Jung B, Jaber S. Intubation in the ICU: we could improve our practice. Crit Care. 2014;18(2):209.
3. De Jong A, Jaber S. Apneic oxygenation for intubation in the critically Ill. Let's not give up! Am J Respir Crit Care Med. 2016;193(3):230–2.
4. Sakles JC, Mosier JM, Patanwala AE, Dicken JM. Apneic oxygenation is associated with a reduction in the incidence of hypoxemia during the RSI of patients with intracranial hemorrhage in the emergency department. Intern Emerg Med. 2016;11(7):983–92.

5. Sakles JC, Mosier JM, Patanwala AE, Arcaris B, Dicken JM, Sakles JC, et al. First pass success without hypoxemia is increased with the use of Apneic oxygenation during rapid sequence intubation in the emergency department. Acad Emerg Med. 2016;23(6):703–10.
6. Semler MW, Janz DR, Lentz RJ, Matthews DT, Norman BC, Assad TR, et al. Randomized trial of Apneic oxygenation during endotracheal intubation of the critically ill. Am J Respir Crit Care Med. 2016;193(3):273–80.
7. Jaber S, Monnin M, Girard M, Conseil M, Cisse M, Carr J, et al. Apnoeic oxygenation via high-flow nasal cannula oxygen combined with non-invasive ventilation preoxygenation for intubation in hypoxaemic patients in the intensive care unit: the single-Centre, blinded, randomised controlled OPTINIV trial. Intensive Care Med. 2016;42(12):1877–87.
8. McQuade D, Miller MR, Hayes-Bradley C. Addition of nasal cannula can either impair or enhance Preoxygenation with a bag valve mask: a randomized crossover design study comparing oxygen flow rates. Anesth Analg. 2018;126(4):1214–8.
9. Ramachandran SK, Cosnowski A, Shanks A, Turner CR. Apneic oxygenation during prolonged laryngoscopy in obese patients: a randomized, controlled trial of nasal oxygen administration. J Clin Anesth. 2010;22(3):164–8.
10. Wong DT, Dallaire A, Singh KP, Madhusudan P, Jackson T, Singh M, et al. High-flow nasal oxygen improves safe apnea time in morbidly obese patients undergoing general anesthesia: a randomized controlled trial. Anesth Analg. 2019;129:1130. Publish Ahead of Print
11. Heinrich S, Horbach T, Stubner B, Prottengeier J, Irouschek A, Schmidt J. Benefits of heated and humidified high flow nasal oxygen for preoxygenation in morbidly obese patients undergoing bariatric surgery: a randomized controlled study. J Obes Bariatrics. 2014;1(1):7.
12. Mir F, Patel A, Iqbal R, Cecconi M, Nouraei SA. A randomised controlled trial comparing transnasal humidified rapid insufflation ventilatory exchange (THRIVE) pre-oxygenation with facemask pre-oxygenation in patients undergoing rapid sequence induction of anaesthesia. Anaesthesia. 2017;72(4):439–43.
13. Lodenius A, Piehl J, Ostlund A, Ullman J, Jonsson FM. Transnasal humidified rapid-insufflation ventilatory exchange (THRIVE) vs. facemask breathing pre-oxygenation for rapid sequence induction in adults: a prospective randomised non-blinded clinical trial. Anaesthesia. 2018;73(5):564–71.
14. Ng I, Krieser R, Mezzavia P, Lee K, Tseng C, Douglas N, et al. The use of Transnasal humidified rapid-insufflation Ventilatory exchange (THRIVE) for pre-oxygenation in neurosurgical patients: a randomised controlled trial. Anaesth Intensive Care. 2018;46(4):360–7.
15. Joseph N, Rajan S, Tosh P, Kadapamannil D, Kumar L. Comparison of arterial oxygenation and Acid-Base balance with the use of Transnasal humidified rapid-insufflation Ventilatory exchange versus tidal volume breathing with continuous positive airway pressure for Preoxygenation and Apneic ventilation. Anesth Essays Res. 2018;12(1):246–50.
16. Tan PCF, Millay OJ, Leeton L, Dennis AT. High-flow humidified nasal preoxygenation in pregnant women: a prospective observational study. Br J Anaesth. 2019;122(1):86–91.
17. Hanouz J-L, Lhermitte D, Gerard J-L, Fischer MO. Comparison of pre-oxygenation using spontaneous breathing through face mask and high-flow nasal oxygen: A prospective randomised crossover controlled study in healthy volunteers. Eur J Anaesthesiol. 2019;36:335. Publish Ahead of Print
18. Patel A, Nouraei SA. Transnasal humidified rapid-insufflation Ventilatory exchange (THRIVE): a physiological method of increasing apnoea time in patients with difficult airways. Anaesthesia. 2015;70(3):323–9.
19. Ebeling CG, Riccio CA. Apneic oxygenation with high-flow nasal cannula and transcutaneous carbon dioxide monitoring during airway surgery: a case series. A A Pract. 2018;12:366.
20. Gustafsson IM, Lodenius A, Tunelli J, Ullman J, Jonsson FM. Apnoeic oxygenation in adults under general anaesthesia using Transnasal humidified rapid-insufflation Ventilatory exchange (THRIVE) - a physiological study. Br J Anaesth. 2017;118(4):610–7.
21. Ffrench-O'Carroll R, Fitzpatrick K, Jonker WR, Choo M, Tujjar O. Maintaining oxygenation with high-flow nasal cannula during emergent awake surgical tracheostomy. Br J Anaesth. 2017;118(6):954–5.

22. Jonker Y, Rutten DJ, van Exel ER, Stek ML, de Bruin PE, Huitink JM. Transnasal humidified rapid-insufflation ventilatory exchange during electroconvulsive therapy: a feasibility study. J ECT. 2018;35:110.
23. Onwochei D, El-Boghdadly K, Oakley R, Ahmad I. Intra-oral ignition of monopolar diathermy during transnasal humidified rapid-insufflation ventilatory exchange (THRIVE). Anaesthesia. 2017;72(6):781–3.
24. Humphreys S, Lee-Archer P, Reyne G, Long D, Williams T, Schibler A. Transnasal humidified rapid-insufflation ventilatory exchange (THRIVE) in children: a randomized controlled trial. Br J Anaesth. 2017;118(2):232–8.
25. Riva T, Pedersen TH, Seiler S, Kasper N, Theiler L, Greif R, et al. Transnasal humidified rapid insufflation ventilatory exchange for oxygenation of children during apnoea: a prospective randomised controlled trial. Br J Anaesth. 2018;120(3):592–9.

Clinical Applications of High-Flow Nasal Cannula in Obstructive Lung Diseases

7

Giulia Spoletini and Lara Pisani

7.1   Introduction

Obstructive lung disease is an umbrella term encompassing respiratory conditions characterized by airflow obstruction secondary to several pathophysiological mechanisms. Obstructive lung diseases include asthma, bronchiectasis, cystic fibrosis, and chronic obstructive pulmonary disease (COPD), and represent one of the major causes of long-term disabilities worldwide.

Oxygen therapy and non-invasive ventilation have been applied in various capacities to the treatment of these conditions both in the acute and chronic setting. Over the last two decades, high-flow nasal therapy (HFNT) has become available as an alternative to deliver respiratory support in a variety of clinical scenarios. By providing high flows of oxygen-enriched gas with low-level positive pressure, HFNT has been suggested as an alternative to conventional oxygen therapy (COT) or to NIV.

To date, most studies have focused on the role of HFNT in patients with acute hypoxaemic respiratory failure or in the critical care unit. However, considering its physiological mechanisms of action, there is a rationale to extend the use of HFNT to obstructive lung disease as well.

In this chapter, we provide a brief overview of this physiological rationale, review and discuss the currently available evidence on the use of HFNT in

G. Spoletini
Respiratory Department, St James's University Hospital, Leeds Teaching Hospital NHS Trust, Leeds, UK

Leeds Institute of Medical Research, University of Leeds, Leeds, UK
e-mail: giulia.spoletini@nhs.net

L. Pisani (✉)
Respiratory and Critical Care Unit, Department of Cardiac-Thoracic and Vascular Diseases, University Hospital St Orsola-Malpighi, Bologna, Italy
e-mail: lara.pisani@aosp.bo.it

© Springer Nature Switzerland AG 2021
A. Carlucci, S. M. Maggiore (eds.), *High Flow Nasal Cannula*,
https://doi.org/10.1007/978-3-030-42454-1_7

obstructive lung disease in the acute and chronic setting, and suggest possible future applications.

7.2 Physiological Mechanisms and Rationale for the Use of HFNT

Airflow obstruction in obstructive lung disease is a consequence of several pathological mechanisms which include various degrees of inflammation with subsequent mucus hypersecretion, collapsible airways and alveoli, parenchymal destruction, and changes in pulmonary mechanics. The latter leads to increased work of breathing, respiratory rate, and dead-space ventilation.

Here we briefly summarize the main physiological mechanisms of action of HFNT that can tackle the above-listed pathological features of obstructive lung disease (Table 7.1).

7.2.1 Effects on Mucociliary Clearance

Mucus hypersecretion and impaired mucociliary clearance in COPD and bronchiectasis are associated with a worsening in the decline of lung function, atelectasis, and pulmonary exacerbations. When patients are treated with COT, devices which provide cold-air humidification, despite being routinely used, do not confer any clinical advantage compared to not providing any humidification [1]; actually the cold and not fully saturated air provided could lead to further airway bronchoconstriction and epithelial desiccation [2].

In contrast, HFNT, by warming the gas to core temperature (37 C) and by fully humidifying it (AH 44 mg/l, RH 100%), preserves the rheology of secretions and provides the airway epithelium with the optimal conditions for ciliary function and mucus transport, with no risk of thermal injuries [2–4]. An acute and short-term exposure to HFNT (3 h) has been shown to improve, but not normalize, lung

Table 7.1 Mechanisms of clinical benefit during HFNT

Mechanism	Effect
Nasal prongs	– Reduced instrumental dead space – Increased comfort
Heating and humidification	– Optimal conditions for: – Mucus rheology properties – Mucociliary clearance – Decreased metabolic cost of breathing
High flow rates	– Inspiratory resistance
Positive airway pressure	– Reduced work of breathing – Reduced respiratory rate – Increased EELV
Washout of functional dead space	– Reduced rebreathing – Increased efficiency of ventilation

mucociliary clearance for a sustained period of time (6 h) in patients with bronchiectasis [4].

7.2.2 Effects on Dead Space

HFNT minimizes the risk of CO_2 rebreathing as an effect of reduced instrumental and functional dead space. Nasal prongs introduce a much lower instrumental dead space compared with any other respiratory interface. Furthermore, by washing out the upper and lower airway dead space, HFNT continuously flushes out CO_2, reducing the F_iCO_2 and increasing the F_iO_2, in a flow-dependent manner, with greater effects shown for flows >30 L/min [5–8].

7.2.3 Effects on Work of Breathing

Patients with obstructive lung disease have inefficient respiratory mechanics, both during wakefulness and sleep. Increased respiratory muscle load, intrinsic PEEP, and increased respiratory rate are among the main mechanisms responsible for a high work of breathing in these conditions [9].

By delivering a positive airway pressure throughout the respiratory cycle [10–13], with a higher pressure at the end of the expiration, HFNT can counterbalance the intrinsic PEEP. This reduces the respiratory muscle load compared to COT, both in sleep and in wakefulness [14, 15].

Furthermore, despite not providing active inspiratory pressure, the ability to attenuate inspiratory resistance contributes to a reduction in respiratory rate [14–16]. This, in conjunction with increases in T_e and subsequent optimization of the I:E, improves ventilatory efficiency and reduces work of breathing [14, 16].

7.3   Potential Clinical Applications

7.3.1 Stable COPD

COPD is the fourth leading cause of morbidity and mortality worldwide [17]. End-stage lung disease is associated with severely impaired quality of life, reduced level of activity, recurrent exacerbations, and hospitalizations. Hypercarbia and chronic respiratory failure are associated with an increased risk of acute deterioration, further decline, and mortality in COPD [18–20].

As COPD is an incurable chronic disease, a major objective in the treatment of this condition is the improvement of quality of life for the affected patients, which can be achieved by improving gas exchange and reducing the rate of exacerbations.

Long-term oxygen therapy (LTOT) was the first treatment shown to improve morbidity and mortality in patients with COPD and chronic respiratory failure [21, 22].

More recently, a growing body of evidence has started supporting a role of NIV in stable COPD, to improve gas exchange and reduce readmission rate, which could ultimately improve the survival rate of patients [23–27].

In view of the mechanisms highlighted above, HFNT can play a role in the integrated management interventions for patients with COPD. We will here discuss the limited available evidence on the effects of HFNT on the quality of life, exacerbation rate, lung function, and gas exchange.

7.3.1.1 Effects on Quality of Life (QoL)

Limitations in daily life and physical activity are among the main determinants of poor quality of life in patients with COPD, and, together with recurrent exacerbations, can lead to increased anxiety and depression. Pharmacological and non-pharmacological approaches have been studied as a means to improve QoL with varying degrees of success [28].

While concerns have been raised about LTOT possibly worsening patients' QoL by restricting their mobility as an effect of their having to carry the equipment and the psychological consequences of the long-term dependency to the treatment, the limited evidence available indicates a positive effect of LTOT on QoL. Beneficial effects have been shown to appear within a relatively short time after the prescription (2 months) and persist in the long term [29].

Similarly, the use of HFNT, with varying F_iO_2 including at 21%, is associated with improvement in QoL as measured by the St George's Respiratory Questionnaire [30–32]. This improvement was observed with both low (1–2 h/day) and more prolonged (6 h/day) use of HFNT in patients with and without chronic respiratory failure. A clinically significant improvement in the SGQR, overall and in each component (5.9–10.8 points), was noted in studies at 3 and 12 months. Interestingly, however, this was not consistently associated with an improvement in exercise capacity as measured by the 6-min walking distance or in lung function. This suggests the presence of other mechanisms underlying the improved QoL and can be related to comfort of the interface, relief of the dyspnoea, reduction in the respiratory rate and work of breathing, and effect on exacerbations.

7.3.1.2 Effects on Exacerbations

Airway surface dehydration plays an important role in COPD by leading to persistent neutrophilic inflammation and mucus hypersecretion [30]. This feeds a vicious cycle linked to recurrent exacerbations and progressive lung damage.

HFNT improves mucociliary clearance by virtue of its effects on mucus properties and optimization of the respiratory epithelium. This can lead to a reduced rate of exacerbation and hospitalization. At the time of writing, only two studies have examined the effects of long-term (1 year) treatment with HFNT in COPD on exacerbations in comparison to standard care. Rea and colleagues compared HFNT at 20 L/min with F_iO_2 0.21 delivered for 1–2 h/day to usual care in patients with moderate COPD and bronchiectasis. Treatment with HFNT was associated with increased time to first exacerbation and reduced number of exacerbation days, but overall similar number of exacerbations [30]. Storgaard and colleagues, more recently, confirmed and expanded these results. Treatment with HFNT at 30 L/min and LTOT was associated with a lower number of exacerbations compared to LTOT alone in patients with COPD and chronic respiratory failure. HFNT was used on average for 6 h/day, but an increased use of HFNT resulted in further reduction of exacerbations [31].

7.3.1.3 Effects on Gas Exchange

Improvement of gas exchange is of the utmost importance in treating patients with COPD, as normalization of the levels of pCO_2 and pO_2 has beneficial effects both physiologically and clinically.

A handful of short-term studies on a small number of patients (ranging from 8 to 77) have shown that delivering high-flow nasal therapy to patients with stable COPD and chronic hypercarbia leads to a significant fall in pCO_2 both during wakefulness and sleep [8, 14–16, 33–35]. Patients were treated with HFNT at flow rates of 15, 20, or 30 L/min, depending on the study, for a time between 30 min and 8 h. A decreased pCO_2 was observed in all studies independently of the flow rate used, with greater effects corresponding to the highest flow of 30 L/min [8, 14, 34]. This flow rate led to a drop in pCO_2 comparable to that observed on NIV [14]. Interestingly, the decline in pCO_2 was not only dependent on the flow rate but also more marked the higher the baseline pCO_2 was, averaging at −10% for a pCO_2 > 50 mmHg [36].

Three recent long-term studies confirmed these results after a period of treatment of 6, 12, and 52 weeks, respectively, with the sustained effect on pCO_2 confirmed also during sleep [31, 32, 37]. In addition, it was shown that the reduction in pCO_2 achieved after 20 minutes of treatment was preserved after 6 and 12 months of continued use (average of 6 h/day) [31].

While results on CO_2 levels are consistent across available studies, evidence on the effect of HFNT on oxygenation is more limited and conflicting. Not all studies reported variables of oxygenation (pO_2 or S_pO_2), with most of them showing no change in oxygenation compared to LTOT both in the short and long term. A single short-term trial using HFNT at 50 L/min for 1 h showed improvement in oxygenation, with reduced F_iO_2 requirements compared to COT [35]. Conversely, a statistically, but possibly not clinically, significant drop in oxygenation was observed during sleep, and in the study comparing HFNT at 30 L/min to COT for a 20-min period [15, 16].

These effects on CO_2 are likely to be correlated with an increase in tidal volume and might be a consequence of dead space and CO_2 washout with assistance of the reduced work of breathing. On the other hand, lower oxygenation on HFNT could mirror a higher F_iO_2 delivered through COT, as under those conditions F_iO_2 cannot be precisely controlled.

7.3.1.4 Other Outcomes

HFNT appears to be safe and well tolerated with no significant side effects experienced by patients who have used it long term. Comfort is generally very good on HFNT, although not consistently across the studies available in the literature.

Tolerability and comfort depended on the delivered flow, and appear to be best at 30 l/min [38].

Limited and conflicting data are available on the effects of HFNT on lung function and 6-min walking test distance and perceived dyspnoea. Preliminary data demonstrate that HFNT may improve exercise performance in patients with advanced COPD and ventilatory limitation by enhancing oxygen saturation and reducing symptoms [39].

However, only one study to date looked at mortality as secondary outcome, and showed no differences in all-cause mortality in patients treated with HFNT compared to LTOT [31].

Despite these promising results, further large multicentre randomized controlled trials comparing HFNT to NIV and COT in the treatment of patients with stable COPD are needed to confirm these results and to further assess the role of HFNT on exacerbations, hospitalization, and survival rates. Until such trials are completed, it is difficult to make a strong practical recommendation to use HFNT in the management of stable patients with COPD. In general, it appears that lower flow rates compared to those used in acute hypoxaemic respiratory failure are sufficient to achieve good outcomes and ensure better tolerability in patients with obstructive lung disease in chronic settings.

7.3.2   Acute Exacerbations of COPD

Severe COPD exacerbation is defined as a sustained worsening of the patient's condition and chronic respiratory symptoms with the onset of acidosis and carbon dioxide retention. When acute hypercapnic respiratory failure occurs, standard medical therapy alone may fail in about 74% of patients [40]. The recent ERS/ATS clinical practice guidelines strongly recommend the application of NIV for patients with ARF leading to acute or acute-on-chronic respiratory acidosis (pH $\leqslant 7.35$) and not in those patients with acute exacerbation of COPD (AECOPD) and hypercapnia who are not acidotic [41]. In fact, NIV can prevent further worsening and clinical deterioration by increasing alveolar ventilation [42 and reducing respiratory effort [43]. At the same time, NIV improves dyspnoea [40, 41, 44], vital signs, and gas exchange [40, 41], and reduces need for intubation [40, 41, 45, 46], hospital length of stay [41, 46], as well as mortality [40, 41, 46].

Although NIV is universally recognized as the gold standard for hypercapnic ARF due to COPD exacerbation, it does not come without some drawbacks. Inappropriately prolonged NIV may delay intubation and ventilation, resulting in worse outcomes [47]. In addition, NIV is not always well tolerated. The interface may be uncomfortable and claustrophobic. Furthermore, success is dependent on patient selection, underlying pathology, and expertise with NIV. In fact, an inadequate level of care is associated with an increased likelihood of NIV failure [48].

In an observational survey conducted in the UK, Roberts et al. [49] showed that one-third of all eligible patients did not receive NIV, while 11% of those with metabolic acidosis did. In addition, mortality was significantly higher in patients treated with NIV than in patients who did not receive NIV with the same level of respiratory acidosis. Although the authors did not specify how many of NIV patients were managed in high-dependency units (HDUs) or intensive care unit (ICUs), this study demonstrated that NIV can be safely administered only in an adequately staffed and monitored unit [48, 49]. Differently, NIV may be harmful by delaying the institution of the appropriate therapy, e.g., invasive ventilation [48, 50].

Whether HFNT might have an impact on hypercapnic ARF is questionable. As mentioned before, from a physiological point of view, the beneficial effects of HFNT include the reduction of dead space and nasopharyngeal resistance [5–8], as well as the improvement of secretion removal [4, 30], and elevation in end-expiratory pressure [10–13]. It also is likely to be better tolerated than NIV [51].

Although physiological short-term studies have shown that HFNT can generate an acute reduction of P_aCO_2 and improve the breathing pattern in stable chronic COPD patients with chronic respiratory failure [14, 16], its role in hypercapnic ARF has not been yet defined, mainly because NIV is strongly recommended as first-line treatment.

Cases of patients with AECOPD and respiratory acidosis successfully treated with HFNT, following interruption of NIV due to poor tolerance, have been reported [52–54].

Additionally, a single-centre randomized controlled crossover trial conducted in 24 AECOPD patients showed that short-term use of HFNT at 35 L/min results in a small reduction in transcutaneous carbon dioxide tension (PtCO2) at 30 min adjusted for time zero compared with standard nasal prongs (-1.4 mm Hg (95% CI: -2.2 to -0.6), $p = 0.001$) [55]. Unfortunately, the authors did not perform ABG at baseline nor did they utilize repeat arterial blood gas sampling, so no information regarding the severity of exacerbation or the pH level is available [55].

Recently, Kim et al. [56] retrospectively investigated the feasibility of the use of HFNT in patients with acute hypercapnic respiratory failure who were admitted to the medical intensive care unit (MICU). Compared to COT, HFNT led to a significant improvement in hypercapnia ($p = 0.006$ and 0.062 after 1 and 24 h, respectively).

In another single-centre prospective trial, Lee and colleagues [57] compared NIV and HFNT in hypercapnic patients with pH between 7.25 and 7.35. The intubation rate (25.0% in the HFNT group and 27.3% in the NIV group) and 30-day mortality (15.9% in the HFNT group and 18.2% in the NIV group, respectively) were not significantly different between two groups. This study also demonstrated a significant decrease in $PaCO_2$ in addition to pH and PaO_2 improvements after 6 and 24 hours of HFNT. However, these results should be interpreted with great caution. The current study, in fact, has several limitations and bias as recognized by the authors, related to the study design, small simple size, and ensuing lack of power [57].

Finally, when specifically addressing the breaks in between NIV sessions, only one RCT has evaluated HFNT in the setting of acute respiratory failure [58]. Out of 47 patients included in the analysis, 22 had an acute or acute-on-chronic hypercapnic respiratory failure, while 25 had hypoxic respiratory failure [58]. In addition, COPD along with arterial hypertension was the most frequent comorbidity.

Interestingly, compared to conventional treatment, HFNT did not reduce the total time spent on NIV or lengthen the time on break. However, it was more tolerated by the patients, causing less eye irritation than standard oxygen [58]. In contrast to standard therapy, HFNT was also able to maintain a steady respiratory rate and level of dyspnoea compared to NIV. The small numbers of patients, the early termination, as well as the fact that both hypoxaemic and hypercapnic patients were included represent some limitations of this study [58].

The ongoing multicentre randomized "HIGH-FLOW ACRF" study [59] will add important information on this topic, focusing on patients with AECOPD. In fact, this trial will assess the hypothesis that HFNT, applied during breaks of NIV, would increase the ventilator-free days and reduce the mortality rate at day 28 in patients with hypercapnic acute respiratory failure compared to standard oxygen.

Taken together, these results suggest a potential for HFNT efficacy in this subgroup of patients not only during breaks of NIV but also when NIV is not or poorly tolerated.

7.3.3 Other Obstructive Lung Diseases

By virtue of its physiological mechanisms on mucociliary clearance [4], it is conceivable that HFNT could exert beneficial effects for patients with other respiratory conditions characterized by mucus hypersecretions and repeated infection, leading eventually to respiratory failure, such as cystic fibrosis (CF) and non-CF bronchiectasis. Less than a handful of reports in abstract form have shown that HFNT is used in clinical practice in CF to facilitate secretion removal and provide at the same time oxygen supplementation. Recently, the first short-term randomized crossover trial compared HFNT to NIV in patients with CF [39] admitted with acute exacerbation, but stabilized with medical treatment and NIV if needed. In this small study ($n = 15$), HFNT had similar effect to NIV on diaphragmatic work per breath as assessed via ultrasound but confers benefits by decreasing respiratory rate and minute ventilation. Interestingly comfort and dyspnoea were similar on HFNT and NIV.

Further trials are needed to explore the potential use of HFNT in patients with CF or non-CF bronchiectasis, both as an adjunct to physiotherapy and in the setting of acute respiratory failure.

7.4   Conclusion

Although the available clinical data for application of HFNT in COPD are increasing over time, there are still some unanswered questions regarding practical aspects of its use. Randomized controlled trials are needed to clarify the real efficacy of HFNT, the best target population, and whether it could be an alternative for patients who cannot tolerate standard NIV and/or could be used during NIV breaks both in the acute and chronic setting.

References

1. Bhowmik A, Chahal K, Austin G, Chakravorty I. Improving mucociliary clearance in chronic obstructive pulmonary disease. Respir Med. 2009;103:496–502.
2. Williams R, Rankin N, Smith T, Galler D, Seakins P. Relationship between the humidity and temperature of inspired gas and the function of the airway mucosa. Crit Care Med. 1996;24:1920–9.
3. Kilgour E, Rankin N, Ryan S, Pack R. Mucociliary function deteriorates in the clinical range of inspired air temperature and humidity. Intensive Care Med. 2004;30:1491–4.
4. Hasani A, Chapman TH, Mccool D, Smith RE, Dilworth JP, Agnew JE. Domiciliary humidification improves lung mucociliary clearance in patients with bronchiectasis. 2008; https://doi.org/10.1177/1479972307087190.
5. Frizzola M, Miller TL, Rodriguez ME, Zhu Y, Rojas J, Hesek A, Stump A, Shaffer TH, Dysart K. High-flow nasal cannula: impact on oxygenation and ventilation in an acute lung injury model. Pediatr Pulmonol. 2011;46:67–74.
6. Möller W, Celik G, Feng S, Bartenstein P, Meyer G, Oliver E, Schmid O, Tatkov S. Nasal high flow clears anatomical dead space in upper airway models. J Appl Physiol. 2015;118:1525–32.
7. Bräunlich J, Wirtz H. Nasal high flow (NHF) reduces PCO2 in a sheep lung model via airway wash-out. Pneumologie. 2016;70:P10.
8. Bräunlich J, Mauersberger F, Wirtz H. Effectiveness of nasal high flow in hypercapnic COPD patients is flow and leakage dependent. BMC Pulm Med. 2018;18:14.
9. Laveneziana P, Guenette JA, Webb KA, O'Donnell DE. New physiological insights into dyspnea and exercise intolerance in chronic obstructive pulmonary disease patients. Expert Rev Respir Med. 2012;6:651–62.
10. Groves N, Tobin A. High flow nasal oxygen generates positive airway pressure in adult volunteers. Aust Crit Care. 2007;20:126–31.
11. Ritchie JEE, Williams AB, Gerard C, Hockey H. Evaluation of humidified nasal high flow oxygen system, using oxygraphy, capnography and measurement of upper airway pressures. Anaesth Intensive Care. 2011;39:1103–10.
12. Parke RL, McGuinness SP. Pressures delivered by nasal high flow oxygen during all phases of the respiratory cycle. Respir Care. 2013;58:1621–4.
13. Parke RL, Eccleston ML, McGuinness SP. The effects of flow on airway pressure during nasal high-flow oxygen therapy. Respir Care. 2011;56:1151–5.
14. Pisani L, Fasano L, Corcione N, Comellini V, Musti MA, Brandao M, Bottone D, Calderini E, Navalesi P, Nava S. Change in pulmonary mechanics and the effect on breathing pattern of high flow oxygen therapy in stable hypercapnic COPD. Thorax. 2017;72:373–5.
15. Biselli PJC, Kirkness JP, Grote L, Fricke K, Schwartz AR, Smith P, Schneider H. Nasal high-flow therapy reduces work of breathing compared with oxygen during sleep in COPD and smoking controls: a prospective observational study. J Appl Physiol. 2017;122:82–8.
16. Fraser JF, Spooner AJ, Dunster KR, Anstey CM, Corley A. Nasal high flow oxygen therapy in patients with COPD reduces respiratory rate and tissue carbon dioxide while increasing tidal and end-expiratory lung volumes: a randomised crossover trial. Thorax. 2016;71:759–61.
17. GBD 2015 Chronic Respiratory Disease Collaborators JB, Abajobir AA, Abate KH, et al. Global, regional, and national deaths, prevalence, disability-adjusted life years, and years lived with disability for chronic obstructive pulmonary disease and asthma, 1990–2015: a systematic analysis for the Global Burden of Disease Study 2015. Lancet Respir Med. 2017;5:691–706.
18. Connors AF, Dawson NV, Thomas C, Harrell FE, Desbiens N, Fulkerson WJ, Kussin P, Bellamy P, Goldman L, Knaus WA. Outcomes following acute exacerbation of severe chronic obstructive lung disease. The SUPPORT investigators (study to understand prognoses and preferences for outcomes and risks of treatments). Am J Respir Crit Care Med. 1996;154:959–67.
19. Murray I, Paterson E, Thain G, Currie GP. Outcomes following non-invasive ventilation for hypercapnic exacerbations of chronic obstructive pulmonary disease. Thorax. 2011;66:825–6.

20. Suh E-S, Mandal S, Harding R, et al. Neural respiratory drive predicts clinical deterioration and safe discharge in exacerbations of COPD. Thorax. 2015;70:1123–30.
21. NOTT Study group. Is 12-hour oxygen as effective as 24-hour oxygen in advanced chronic obstructive pulmonary disease with hypoxemia? (the nocturnal oxygen therapy trial—NOTT). Chest. 1980;78:419–20.
22. NOTT Study Group. Continuous or nocturnal oxygen therapy in hypoxemic chronic obstructive lung disease: a clinical trial. Nocturnal oxygen therapy trial group. Ann Intern Med. 1980;93:391–8.
23. Elliott MW, Mulvey DA, Moxham J, Green M, Branthwaite MA. Domiciliary nocturnal nasal intermittent positive pressure ventilation in COPD: mechanisms underlying changes in arterial blood gas tensions. Eur Respir J. 1991;4:1044–52.
24. Meecham Jones DJ, Paul EA, Jones PW, Wedzicha JA. Nasal pressure support ventilation plus oxygen compared with oxygen therapy alone in hypercapnic COPD. Am J Respir Crit Care Med. 1995;152:538–44.
25. Nickol A, Hart N, Hopkinson NS, Hamnegård C-H, Moxham J, Simonds A, Polkey MI. Mechanisms of improvement of respiratory failure in patients with COPD treated with NIV. Int J Chron Obstruct Pulmon Dis. 2008;3:453–62.
26. Köhnlein T, Windisch W, Köhler D, et al. Non-invasive positive pressure ventilation for the treatment of severe stable chronic obstructive pulmonary disease: a prospective, multicentre, randomised, controlled clinical trial. Lancet Respir Med. 2014;2:698–705.
27. Murphy PB, Rehal S, Arbane G, et al. Effect of home noninvasive ventilation with oxygen therapy vs oxygen therapy alone on hospital readmission or death after an acute COPD exacerbation. JAMA. 2017;317:2177.
28. Brien SB, Lewith GT, Thomas M. Patient coping strategies in COPD across disease severity and quality of life: a qualitative study. NPJ Prim Care Respir Med. 2016;26:16051.
29. Eaton T, Lewis C, Young P, Kennedy Y, Garrett J, Kolbe J. Long-term oxygen therapy improves health-related quality of life. Respir Med. 2004;98:285–93.
30. Rea H, McAuley S, Jayaram L, Garrett J, Hockey H, Storey L, O'Donnell G, Haru L, Payton M, O'Donnell K. The clinical utility of long-term humidification therapy in chronic airway disease. Respir Med. 2010;104:525–33.
31. Storgaard LH, Hockey H, Laursen BS, Weinreich UM. Long-term effects of oxygen-enriched high-flow nasal cannula treatment in COPD patients with chronic hypoxemic respiratory failure. Int J Chron Obstruct Pulmon Dis. 2018;13:1195–205.
32. Nagata K, Kikuchi T, Horie T, et al. Domiciliary high-flow nasal cannula oxygen therapy for patients with stable Hypercapnic chronic obstructive pulmonary disease. A Multicenter randomized crossover trial. Ann Am Thorac Soc. 2018;15:432–9.
33. Braunlich J, Beyer D, Mai D, et al. Effects of nasal high flow in ventilation in volunteers, COPD and idiopathic pulmonary fibrosis patients. Respiration. 2012;85:319–25.
34. Bräunlich J, Köhler M, Wirtz H. Nasal high flow improves ventilation in patients with COPD. Int J Chron Obstruct Pulmon Dis. 2016;11:1077–85.
35. Vogelsinger H, Halank M, Braun S, Wilkens H, Geiser T, Ott S, Stucki A, Kaehler CM. Efficacy and safety of nasal high-flow oxygen in COPD patients. BMC Pulm Med. 2017;17:143.
36. Bräunlich J, Wirtz H. NHF and hypercapnia: how brief can you look? Respirology. 2017;22:1049–50.
37. Bräunlich J, Seyfarth H-J, Wirtz H. Nasal high-flow versus non-invasive ventilation in stable hypercapnic COPD: a preliminary report. Multidiscip Respir Med. 2015;10:27.
38. McKinstry S, Pilcher J, Bardsley G, Berry J, Van de Hei S, Braithwaite I, Fingleton J, Weatherall M, Beasley R. Nasal high flow therapy and PtCO$_2$ in stable COPD: a randomized controlled cross-over trial. Respirology. 2018;23:378–84.
39. Cirio S, Piran M, Vitacca M, Piaggi G, Ceriana P, Prazzoli M, et al. Effects of heated and humidified highflow gases during high-intensity constant-load exercise on severe COPD patients with ventilatory limitation. Respir Med. 2016;118:128–32.
40. Plant PK, Owen JL, Elliott MW. Early use of non-invasive ventilation for acute exacerbations of chronic obstructive pulmonary disease on general respiratory wards: a multicentre randomised controlled trial. Lancet. 2000;355:1931–35.

41. Rochwerg B, Brochard L, Elliott MW, et al. Official ERS/ATS clinical practice guidelines: noninvasive ventilation for acute respiratory failure. Eur Respir J. 2017;50.
42. Diaz O, Iglesia R, Ferrer M, et al. Effects of noninvasive ventilation on pulmonary gas exchange and hemodynamics during acute hypercapnic exacerbations of chronic obstructive pulmonary disease. Am J Respir Crit Care Med. 1997;156:1840–45.
43. Appendini L, Patessio A, Zanaboni S, et al. Physiologic effects of positive end-expiratory pressure and mask pressure support during exacerbations of chronic obstructive pulmonary disease. Am J Respir Crit Care Med. 1994;149:1069–76.
44. Bott J, Carroll MP, Conway JH, et al. Randomised controlled trial of nasal ventilation in acute ventilatory failure due to chronic obstructive airways disease. Lancet. 1993;341:1555–57.
45. Brochard L, Mancebo J, Wysocki M, et al. Noninvasive ventilation for acute exacerbations of chronic obstructive pulmonary disease. N Engl J Med. 1995;333:817–22.
46. Kramer N, Meyer TJ, Meharg J, et al Randomized, prospective trial of noninvasive positive pressure ventilation in acute respiratory failure. Am J Respir Crit Care Med. 1995;151:1799–1806.
47. Ambrosino N, Foglio K, Rubini F, et al. Non-invasive mechanical ventilation in acute respiratory failure due to chronic obstructive airways disease: correlates for success. Thorax. 1995;50:755–57.
48. Ergan B, Nasiłowski J, Winck JC. How should we monitor patients with acute respiratory failure treated with noninvasive ventilation? Eur Respir Rev. 2018;13;27(148).
49. Roberts CM, Stone RA, Buckingham RJ, et al. Acidosis, non-invasive ventilation and mortality in hospitalised COPD exacerbations. Thorax; 2011;66: 43–8.
50. Demoule A, Girou E, Richard JC, et al. Benefits and risks of success or failure of noninvasive ventilation. Intensive Care Med. 2006;32:1756–65.
51. Bräunlich J, Seyfarth HJ, Wirtz H. Nasal high-flow versus non-invasive ventilation in stable hypercapnic COPD: a preliminary report. Multidiscip Respir Med. 2015;10:27.
52. Millar J, Lutton S, O'Connor P. The use of high-flow nasal oxygen therapy in the management of hypercarbic respiratory failure. Ther Adv Respir Dis. 2014;8:63–4.
53. Lepere V, Messika J, La Combe B, et al. High-flow nasal cannula oxygen supply as treatment in hypercapnic respiratory failure. Am J Emerg Med. 2016;34:1914.
54. Plotnikow G, Thille AW, Vasquez D, Pratto R, Desmery P. High-flow nasal cannula oxygen for reverting severe acute exacerbation of chronic obstructive pulmonary disease: A case report. Med Intensiva. 2017;41(9):571–72.
55. Pilcher J, Eastlake L, Richards M, Power S, Cripps T, Bibby S, Braithwaite I, Weatherall M, Beasley R. Physiological effects of titrated oxygen via nasal high-flow cannulae in COPD exacerbations: A randomized controlled cross-over trial. Respirology. 2017;22(6):1149–55.
56. Kim ES, Lee H, Kim SJ, Park J, Lee YJ, Park JS, Yoon HI, Lee JH, Lee CT, Cho YJ. J. Effectiveness of high-flow nasal cannula oxygen therapy for acute respiratory failure with hypercapnia. Thorac Dis. 2018;10(2):882–88.
57. Lee MK, Choi J, Park B, Kim B, Lee SJ, Kim SH, Yong SJ, Choi EH, Lee WY. High flow nasal cannulae oxygen therapy in acute-moderate hypercapnic respiratory failure. Clin Respir J. 2018;12(6):2046–56.
58. Spoletini G, Mega C, Pisani L, Alotaibi M, Khoja A, Price LL, Blasi F, Nava S, Hill NS. High-flow nasal therapy vs standard oxygen during breaks off noninvasive ventilation for acute respiratory failure: A pilot randomized controlled trial. J Crit Care. 2018;48:418–25.
59. Ricard JD, Dib F, Esposito-Farese M, Messika J, Girault C; REVA network. Comparison of high flow nasal cannula oxygen and conventional oxygen therapy on ventilatory support duration during acute-on-chronic respiratory failure: study protocol of a multicentre, randomised, controlled trial. The 'HIGH-FLOW ACRF' study. BMJ Open. 2018;8(9):e022983.

Clinical Applications of High-Flow Nasal Cannula in Pulmonary Rehabilitation

8

Barbara Fusar Poli, Cinzia Lastoria, and Annalisa Carlucci

8.1 Pathophysiology of Exercise Limitation

Chronic respiratory diseases are associated to exertional dyspnoea and limitation to physical activity of a different extent according to the degree of functional impairment. Chronic obstructive pulmonary disease (COPD) represents the prototype of the underlying pathophysiological mechanisms. Exercise limitation in this respiratory disease is multifactorial. Lung function, inspiratory and peripheral muscle force and age, among others, have been shown to be important determinants of exercise capacity [1]. Cardiovascular disease is a frequent comorbidity in COPD, due to the high prevalence of smoking and other known risk factors such as poor diet, a sedentary lifestyle and systemic inflammation. Moreover, mild-to-moderate pulmonary hypertension is a common complication of COPD. These comorbidities also contribute to the limitation of exercise performance [1]. In this chapter we focus on the main mechanisms involved in the ventilatory limitation that is one important cause of exertional dyspnoea. Some of these mechanisms may be responsive to the use of high-flow nasal cannula (HFNC). The main respiratory causes of ventilatory limitation in a typical COPD patient are shown in Fig. 8.1. The reduction of forced expiratory volume at the first second (FEV1), due to the increased expiratory resistances and the decreased elastic recoil of the lung, causes a reduction of the maximal ventilatory capacity that is the maximal increase of the minute ventilation the patient could reach during the effort (Fig. 8.2). However, the reduction of FEV1 is not the only determinant of exercise limitation, so that this parameter cannot predict the level of performance to exercise [2]. During the effort, the expiratory flow limitation and the progressive increase of respiratory rate may result in a progressive increase of the end-expiratory lung volume (EELV), leading to both a dynamic hyperinflation and the increase of the intrinsic positive end-expiratory pressure

B. Fusar Poli · C. Lastoria · A. Carlucci (✉)
Pulmonary Rehabilitation, Istituti Clinici Scientifici Maugeri, Pavia, Italy
e-mail: annalisa.carlucci@icsmaugeri.it

© Springer Nature Switzerland AG 2021
A. Carlucci, S. M. Maggiore (eds.), *High Flow Nasal Cannula*,
https://doi.org/10.1007/978-3-030-42454-1_8

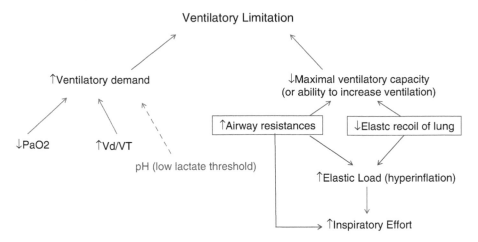

Fig. 8.1 Pathophysiological mechanisms responsible for ventilatory limitation. *Vd* dead-space volume, *VT* tidal volume

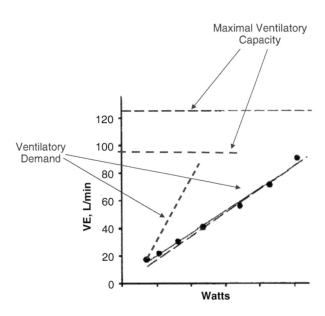

Fig. 8.2 Relation between the variation of minute ventilation (V_E) and workload in COPD (dotted red line) and normal patients (dotted black line)

(PEEPi). The progressive increase of EELV, coupled with the increased tidal breath due to the effort, brings the inspiratory volume close to the total lung capacity [3]. This unfavourable position on the pressure-volume curve of the respiratory system, associated to the dynamic development of PEEPi, leads to a significant increase of the work of breathing and it limits the further increase of tidal volume in spite of the patient's inspiratory requirement, causing a neuro-ventilatory uncoupling and, consequently, dyspnoea [4]. The increase of WOB may switch off the blood flow from limbs to respiratory muscles, leading to earlier peripheral muscle fatigue that may be another reason for exercise interruption. How fast the patient reaches the maximal ventilatory capacity and, consequently, the inability to continue the exercise depends also on the slope of the minute ventilation rise (Fig. 8.2). In COPD patients the ventilatory demand during an incremental test increases during effort when compared to a normal subject at iso-work rate. The reasons for increased ventilatory demand are multiple: the development of hypoxia, production of lactates and increase of dead space. A physiological study showed that an increased dead space is one of the major determinants of dyspnoea and exercise limitation also in mild COPD [5]. This results in compensatory increase in minute ventilation and consequently earlier mechanical constraints on tidal volume leading to a rapid attainment of maximal ventilator capacity (Fig. 8.2).

8.2   Mechanism of Action of High-Flow Nasal Cannula on Exercise Limitation

Nowadays, because of the lack of physiological studies, it is still unclear how the HFNC works during effort, but it is possible to speculate on that. HFNC may influence the mechanisms leading to the excessive increase of ventilation demand during effort in the respiratory disease.

Bräunlich et al. [6] in 2016 showed how HFNC leads to a flow-dependent reduction in PCO_2, obtained principally by a washout of the respiratory tract and by a *functional reduction in dead space*. Patients supported by HFNC modify their breathing pattern by increasing tidal volume and decreasing respiratory rate and, therefore, minute volume while keeping constant or reducing PCO_2. This leads to an improvement of efficiency of ventilation and results in a reduction of the work of breathing. These findings have been shown in COPD patients at rest but it is likely that the same mechanisms may have a role even during exercise, especially in those respiratory diseases where exercise may be associated to an increase of dead-space ventilation; as above-mentioned, it happens in COPD patients also in an early stage of the disease [5]. We already know from bench studies that the level of clearance of upper airways increases proportionally to the set flow used [7]. However, in a recent physiological study on stable hypercapnic COPD patients, Braulinch et al. [8] compared same levels of flow in two different conditions: with and without nose leakages. Authors showed that the higher the leakages, the higher the decrease of PCO_2, despite an associated reduction of mean airway pressure. They concluded that higher flow rates and increased leakage of the upper airways might increase the effectiveness of dead-space washout, and that an increase in airway pressure is not required for this aim.

Another possible benefit on the exercise in respiratory diseases may be the ability of HFNC to guarantee a *better oxygenation*. This may be due to the high dependence of delivered FiO_2 on the patient's inspiratory flow rate when using the majority of oxygen delivery systems [9]. HFNC can generate flow exceeding the patient's peak inspiratory flow rate during effort, keeping constant the delivered FiO_2. Furthermore, the continuous flushing of the nasopharyngeal spaces with "fresh gases" enriched of O2 causes the upper airways to act as a reservoir of O2 [10]. These mechanisms may delay the attainment of ventilator limitation by reducing the slope of minute ventilation increase during the effort [11]. Moreover, the reduction of the ventilatory request leads to a decrease in oxygen cost of breathing and metabolic unloading (reduced lactate production) which may contribute to a further delay of the patient exhaustion [11, 12] and possibly of leg fatigue. However, different mechanisms other than the ability of HFNC to keep constant the delivered FiO_2 seem to be related to a better oxygenation during effort. In fact in a recent study Cirio and co-workers showed that a subgroup of patients making the endurance test at a FiO_2 of 21% had a better oxygen saturation at iso-time when using HFNC than without it [12].

For this reason authors speculated that another mechanism probably involved in the improvement of exercise symptoms is the mild *increase of mean expiratory airway pressure* during expiration. HFNC was showed to increase resistance to expiratory air, causing an increase in peak expiratory pressure (PEP) during the expiratory phase proportional to the delivered flow and to the patient's expiratory flow (progressively increasing during effort) and dependent on the ability of the patient to keep the mouth closed [13, 14]. The increased expiratory resistances may be assimilated to the pursed-lip breathing adopted by the COPD patient to prolong their expiratory time and alleviate expiratory flow limitation and dynamic hyperinflation. The rise in pressure is due to the increase in expiratory resistance due to the delivered flow, but it depends also on the size of the cannula used: the larger the size, the higher the ability to increase the pharyngeal expiratory pressure. PEP effect may counterbalance the auto-PEEP generated by the dynamic hyperinflation during the effort, but may also increase the driving pressure [7]. In fact, in an in vitro model of nasal cavity, Mundel [13] showed that while during spontaneous breathing the inspiratory pressure in the nasal cavity becomes negative with the onset of inspiration, during HFNC delivery the pressure at the onset of inspiration remained above atmosphere for most of the inspiratory phase. This mechanism might have a further role during exercise by *increasing the driving pressure during inspiration.*

Given the findings by Braulinch and Mundel, further studies are needed to understand if it is more useful to favour the expiratory peak pressure by using the highest flow tolerated and avoiding leakages with a cannula size well fitted with the nostrils of the patient and closed mouth, or to favour the best clearance of dead space possible, with high flows and more leakages through the nostrils.

The above-mentioned mechanism of action of HFNC during exercise may be of interest also in patients with systolic heart failure where exercise limitation is not completely explained by cardiac dysfunction.

An Australian study, published in 2016 [15], showed that exercise limitation in left heart failure may be related to the development of excessive dead-space ventilation whose pulmonary diffusing capacity's impairment might be a strong predictor. In fact, in patients with heart failure peripheral pulmonary vasculopathy brings to vascular remodelling, associated with reduced diffusing capacity of the lung for carbon monoxide (DLCO). Decreased DLCO strongly correlates with peak exercise oxygen uptake, heart failure severity class and prognosis but the relationship between reduced DLCO and reduced exercise capacity is unclear, because patients with heart failure rarely have significant oxygen haemoglobin desaturation or falls in arterial oxygen tension with exercise.

Kee and colleagues [15] compared 87 patients affected by heart failure undergoing heart transplant assessment with control group data (18 healthy subjects with normal cardiopulmonary exercise tests). Airway disease, emphysema, pulmonary embolism and right-to-left shunt were excluded. During a maximal incremental cardiopulmonary exercise test, respiratory and metabolic data were collected. Dead-space ventilation at maximum exercise (DSmax) was defined as the proportion of tidal ventilation made up of dead space (anatomical and alveolar dead space) calculated at peak exercise using the Bohr equation. Only patients with heart failure (not controls) showed, at rest, a reduction of DLCO, which was associated with the development of higher dead-space ventilation during exercise with a consequent inefficient ventilation and reduced exercise tolerance. This is the first study proving the relationship between DLCO and DSmax, but also that the increased dead-space ventilation during exercise is caused by ventilation-perfusion mismatch. Anatomical dead space may increase as a percentage of total ventilation when either tidal volume is low or respiratory frequency is high. The study demonstrated that the volume of dead space per breath increased with increasing work, especially in the heart failure group. Since the volume of anatomical dead space per breath is mostly fixed (or is unlikely to increase) during exercise, this fact suggests that alveolar dead space is augmented throughout exercise in this subgroup of patients. Thus the reduced ability to match pulmonary perfusion with ventilation and a consequent increase in dead-space ventilation are present in heart failure patients and probably worsen during exercise. These physiopathological behaviours may represent a rationale for the use of HFNC during effort even in this subgroup of patients.

8.3   Clinical Studies

Patients affected by respiratory diseases, particularly COPD patients, are prone to physical inactivity compared to age-matched healthy individuals [16], with a substantial decrease over time. Physical inactivity independently predicts poor outcomes [17]. Medical literature has firmly affirmed the usefulness of pulmonary rehabilitation in respiratory diseases, in particular in COPD patients, in which it keeps the greatest positive effect of any other current therapy on exercise capacity [18]. The intensity of physical exercise is crucial to achieve a true physiologic effect. However these patients are frequently unable to sustain a workload high enough to obtain full benefits from the training program [19]. For this reason, the addition of different tools has been proposed to improve exercise tolerance during pulmonary rehabilitation, as hyperoxic gas mixture and non-invasive ventilation. However, the above-mentioned treatments are finalised to impact only one mechanism subtending ventilatory limitation.

In the 1990s, some studies compared the effect of low vs. high flow of non-humidified oxygen administered through transtracheal or nasal prongs. The first trial

[20] was conducted in ten COPD patients who performed a modified incremental test with treadmill in four different conditions: two tests receiving low-flow and high-flow transtracheal oxygen (TTO) and the other two with low- and high-flow oxygen by nasal prongs (NP). Mean oxygen flow rates used for low flow were 1.05 ± 0.61 L/min and 1.62 ± 1.3 L/min, whereas mean high flow rates were 5.1 ± 1.64 L/min and 5.9 ± 1.91 L/min, with TTO and NP, respectively. They found that the mean distance, dyspnoea score, oxygen saturation (SpO2) and heart rate were significantly greater with high-flow oxygen (both with TTO and NP) as compared with low-flow oxygen. In particular, mean exercise distance with high-flow TTO was 2.5 times greater than with low-flow TTO, and high flow with NP was 2.38 times greater than low flow ($p < 0.05$). No difference in the end points was found when comparing high flow via TTO and via NP, suggesting that high-flow supplemental oxygen may improve exercise tolerance irrespective of the way of administration.

Some years later, a physiological study aimed to compare the acute effect of supplemental hyperoxic mixture with ambient air during exercise was performed in 11 COPD patients with chronic respiratory failure [21]. Authors found a significant improvement in the endurance time, primarily related to reduced ventilatory demand, which, in turn, led to improved operational lung volumes and a delay in the attainment of ventilatory limitation and the onset of intolerable dyspnoea. Despite several studies in favour of using supplemental oxygen, a Cochrane review concluded for a little support on the use of oxygen therapy during exercise training on COPD patients [22]. The main reasons were the few randomised studies, wide differences in enrollment criteria, small sample size, study design and main end points.

Recently, a randomised, single-blind, crossover study [23], performed on 124 COPD patients, compared the effects of low-flow oxygen to ambient air by stratifying the patients' functional impairment into three groups: patients with normoxia, with exercise-induced hypoxia and with resting hypoxia. They found that only the latter two significantly improved the endurance time with oxygen. However, the response to oxygen was not homogeneous and only half of these patients reached the threshold of clinically relevant improvement.

Apart from the limited support from the literature, the use of oxygen therapy during exercise presents some intrinsic limits because of its dry gas nature leading to nasal dryness, crusting and epistaxis, which appear more frequently with the use of high flows of non-humidified oxygen [24] and may affect the tolerance and adherence to its use during training. Furthermore, in several patients a significant oxygen desaturation may occur, despite the use of high-flow O2. This is due to the entrainment of room air since the rate of patient inspiratory flow during effort easily exceeds the total delivered oxygen flow.

To overcome all the above-described limitations, in 2004, Chatila et al. [25] evaluated the physiological effects of humidified high-flow oxygen (HFO) during exercise in 10 pts. with severe COPD, in comparison to conventional low-flow oxygen (LFO) delivery. The respiratory pattern and work of breathing were measured in both conditions.

Patients were asked to exercise up to 12 min, or less if not tolerated, on unloaded cycle ergometer (that is not the gold standard test to study the efficacy of a treatment), receiving LFO firstly and then HFO in a non-randomised order, after a period of rest of 30 minutes. In both tests, O2 was administered at the expiratory end of a flow transducer put on the mouth and an O2 analyser. Flow and FiO2 were previously titrated, when possible, or arbitrarily chosen with a flow between 2.5 and 6 L/min. The HFO system was adjusted to deliver a total flow of 20 L/min of humidified gas, warmed to 36 °C, and a same FiO_2 measured at rest during LFO administration. However an increase of FiO2 was allowed if a SaO2 < 90% was reached during the tests. During exercise, three patients in LFO had their oxygen flow increase due to Spo2 < 90% (from 30 to 56% of FiO2); this adjustment was not necessary in HFO group. Patients were able to exercise longer with HFO compared to LFO (10.0 ± 2.4 min vs. 8.2 ± 4.3 min, p 0.05), with significantly less dyspnoea and lower mean arterial pressure and heart rate. At iso-time, respiratory rate and Ti/Tot were significantly lower during HFO while no difference in tidal volume and work of breathing was recorded. Surprisingly, minute ventilation did not differ between the two treatments, too. Despite the equivalent FiO2 given at rest, oxygenation and PaO2 were better during HFO ($p = 0.04$ and 0.05, respectively), while pH and PaCO2 were not different. The better oxygenation was considered the most important explanation of the improved exercise tolerance, not adding anything more to the oldest studies comparing low and high non-humidified flow oxygen. The study design presented several limitations: first of all it is a non-randomised study design; COPD patients were enrolled regardless of the documented exercise limitation; a flow of 20 L/min was used, while we know that some physiological effects of HFO are flow dependent; the administration of HFO through the mouth is not suitable to the real life and loses the important effect of dead-space washout. A more recent single-centre crossover study [12] tried to overcome the limits of the previous study by optimising the use of HFNC on 12 stable severe COPD.

A main selection criterion was the exercise limitation defined as a 6-min walk distance <75% of the predicted value. All possible confounding factors were excluded (recent COPD exacerbation, recent change in medication status, left heart failure, neuromuscular disease or osteoarticular limitation).

A symptom-limited incremental exercise test on cycle ergometer was used to set the load for the following endurance tests and to titrate a FiO2 able to reach a mean SaO2 > 88%, subsequently used for the endurance tests. In the following 2 days, two constant-load exercise tests with HFNC (HFNC-test) and with oxygen or ambient air (control test), at iso-FiO2, were randomly performed. The endurance time, SaO2, heart rate, blood pressure, Borg scale for dyspnoea (Borg-D) and leg fatigue (Borg-F) were recorded every minute during the tests.

Four patients performed the two tests on ambient air, while the other eight needed a mean FiO2 of 44 ± 11% administered by a Venturi mask. During the HFNC test, the flow was set at the highest rate tolerated by the patient (mean of 58.7 L/min). The endurance time was significantly higher during the HFNC test (mean difference of 109 ± 104 s, $p < 0.015$). At iso-time, Borg-D and Borg-F were significantly lower while SpO2 was significantly higher during HFNC test ($p < 0.005$).

Interestingly, a significantly higher SpO2 at iso-time during HFNC test was also recorded in the subgroup of patients who made the two constant-load tests in ambient air. Taking into account the very low sample size, this data may confirm that the improvement of exercise tolerance is not only due to a better oxygenation guaranteed, but also due to the high flows matching or even overcoming the inspiratory flow of the patients. Other mechanisms, not dependent on the supplemental oxygen, may be involved. Unfortunately, in this study no measures of breathing pattern, operating volumes and work of breathing were performed to better understand why during HFNC test patients are able to prolong the exercise.

Similar data were reproduced in a South American study that until now has only been published in the form of abstract [26]. The study aimed to compare the exercise tolerance and the comfort to the device of 28 COPD patients by using HFNC or Venturi mask (VM). Patients were asked to perform an incremental exercise test with treadmill and a constant-load test in two different days in a random order with HFNC (with a fixed FiO2 40%, and a fixed flow of 50 L/m) and with VM with the same FiO2. Four dropouts were recorded for exacerbation between the tests. The recorded maximum speed (km/h) in the incremental test was significantly higher in HFNC group (5.9 vs. 5.7 km/h, respectively; $p < 0.001$). The endurance time in the constant-load test was 450 sec in HFNC vs. 315 s in VM group ($p < 0.05$). SpO2 was significantly higher and dyspnoea score significantly lower ($p < 0.05$) both at iso-work and iso-time during HFNC. Leg fatigue, SpO2, heart rate, respiratory rate, blood pressure and comfort were not significantly different.

These two latter studies suggest that the use of HFNC may improve exercise tolerance in COPD patients with a documented exercise limitation in a stable phase of their natural history. Exacerbations are frequently accompanied by a further dramatic daily activity limitation that, in turn, significantly impact the risk of a new exacerbation and death. Early pulmonary rehabilitation was showed to reduce this risk.

However, patients are frequently unable to sustain a workload intensity sufficiently high to guarantee a successful training outcome. Previous studies showed that HFNC may improve toleration of required training intensity.

An ongoing single-centre trial [27], started in April 2017 and with an expected duration of 2 years, has been published as a protocol by a French group. It is aimed to evaluate a possible acute effect of HFNC on endurance time in COPD patients just after a severe exacerbation. HFNC, set up to 60 L/min, is compared to oxygen or room air in two constant-load tests performed in two different days. One first constant-load test is performed at 80% of the peak work rate (estimated by the best of two 6MWT) to titrate both the work rate (the endurance time should be not less than 5 min or more than 15 min) and the oxygen flow able to keep SaO2 > 90% during the exercise (when needed). The oxygen flow titrated is used at the same rate during the test with HFNC and during the test with oxygen by using nasal cannula. Consequently, the two constant-load tests will not be performed at the same FiO2. Primary outcome will be the endurance time. Secondary outcomes will be the evaluation of impact of HFNC on peripheral muscle oxygenation of the right quadriceps muscle, evaluated by spectroscopy in the near-infrared, dyspnoea and muscle fatigue, transcutaneous CO2 pressure, respiratory rate, cardiac rate, SpO2 and respiratory muscle fatigue (evaluated by three measures of maximal inspiratory and expiratory pressure, before and after each test). The calculated sample size is of 19 patients.

Recently, a multicentric randomised-controlled study was published exploring this issue [28], The study enrolled 171 COPD patients with chronic respiratory failure, undergoing a training program with high-intensity exercise. The training consisted of at least 20 cycle ergometer sessions lasting 30 min each, within a 1-month time period (5 sessions per week). Patients were randomised to receive HFNC, using the AIRVO2® device (Fisher&Paykel - Auckland- New Zealand) with a flow at the highest value tolerated and Oxygen with Venturi mask with the same FiO2 set during the runin session. Primary aim was the effort tolerance defined with the endurance time. Several secondary outcomes were also considered, including effectiveness in functional capacity (measured by the 6 Minute Walking Distance), dyspnea at rest, peripheral and respiratory muscle strength, blood gases, and patients' satisfaction. As compared with Venturi-mask, addition of HFNC during exercise training sessions is more effective in improving exercise capacity as assessed by 6MWD but not by endurance time. However, patients presenting a FEV1>30% and an higher baseline endurance time were shown to be possible responder to HFOT.

One of the most important limitations of the use of HFNC during exercise is the lack of an internal battery allowing the use of this potentially useful device only in a protected environment and in a very rigid setting as the use of treadmill or bicycle. An Italian group performed a recent randomised crossover trial to test the feasibility during walking of HFNC, powered by an external battery. The study was published in the form of abstract [29]. Thirteen severe stable COPD patients with a walking distance lower than 70% of predicted and a modified Borg dyspnoea ≥ 5 at 6-minute walk test (6MWT) were enrolled to perform two consecutive 6MWTs: with HFNC and with Venturi mask at the same FiO2 previously titrated in the run-in session. Authors found that walking distance was significantly higher using HFNC, with a median of 306 mt, compared to 267mt performed with Venturi mask ($p < 0.001$). No significant differences were found between the two groups in dyspnoea score and comfort in the device use that showed only a trend to a better confidence with HFNC versus Venturi mask (57 ± 22 mm vs. 40 ± 26 mm to a visual analogue scale). No other significant differences were recorded in the other secondary outcomes: mean SaO2, and change in respiratory rate and in inspiratory capacity.

If several data are coming about the usefulness of HFNC during training of COPD patients, little data are available about its application on other respiratory diseases. Some chronic lung diseases leading to severe hypoxaemia, such as interstitial pulmonary fibrosis (IPF) or pulmonary hypertension, may benefit from a training programme even if the improvement of dyspnoea and exercise capacity might be less consistent and of shorter duration compared to COPD patients [30, 31]. However, the rapid and very severe oxygen desaturation even with oxygen supplement with high FiO2 compromises the ability to keep a certain workload for a time sufficient to make the training session effective to improve exercise tolerance, even during interval training programmes. Apart from the pathophysiology of these respiratory diseases leading to severe hypoxaemia during exercise, another important problem is the inability to guarantee the FiO2 given with the Venturi mask, evident in a higher extent with these patients. In fact, the highest is the FiO2 needed during the effort and the lowest is the total flow that the Venturi system is able to provide. Consequently, the rapid increase of the patient inspiratory flow easily overpasses the total flow delivered by the mask leading to an entrainment of room air and a decrease of FiO2. HFNC can be delivered with a flow of up to 60 L/min and potentially reduce this effect. In particular, data from literature show that the quality of life of IPF patients is markedly limited by severe exertional hypoxaemia, often refractory, for the above-mentioned reasons, to even high rate of supplemental oxygen. Moreover new anti-fibrotic agents may prolong the benefits of exercise training by reducing IPF progression [32, 33]. By now, no data are available in the literature about the use of HFNC for training of hypoxaemic lung diseases.

8.4 Conclusions and Future Applications

Although in the literature until now there are no strong data on the hypothetical use of HFNC to improve activity performance in patients with exercise limitation, from the above-mentioned published and ongoing studies it is possible to speculate a possible role of HFNC both in patients suffering from respiratory diseases (above all COPD, even after a severe exacerbation) and in those suffering from heart diseases with a reduction of pulmonary diffusing lung capacity.

There is still a lack of information about the possible mechanisms by which HFNC may improve effort. Physiological studies are needed to better understand how HFNC may operate and this is very important to better titrate and use HFNC for this aim. We showed, in fact, that the dead-space washout is flow dependent and may be increased by creating a lot of leakages to pharyngeal pressure disadvantage that would increase less in this condition. On the contrary, the increase in expiratory resistances is already flow dependent, but at the same flow rate more increased by fitting well the nasal prongs with the nostrils and minimising the leaks.

Moreover, a complete absence of knowledge regards the possible application of HFNC on very severe hypoxic lung disease during pulmonary rehabilitation. Finally, a technical improvement of the systems used to deliver HFNC is needful to make them transportable (i.e., built-in battery and trolley) to extend the use of them.

References

1. McNamara RJ, Houben-Wilke S, Franssen FME, Smid DE, Vanfleteren LEGW, Groenen MTJ, et al. Determinants of functional, peak and endurance exercise capacity in people with chronic obstructive pulmonary disease. Respir Med. 2018;138:81–7.
2. Gosselink R, Troosters T, Decramer M. Peripheral muscle weakness contributes to exercise limitation in COPD. Am J Respir Crit Care Med. 1996;153(3):976–80.

3. O'Donnell DE, Revill SM, Webb KA. Dynamic hyperinflation and exercise intolerance in chronic obstructive pulmonary disease. Am J Respir Crit Care Med. 2001;164:770–7.
4. Marin JM, Carrizo SJ, Gascon M, Sanchez A, Gallego B, Celli BR. Inspiratory capacity, dynamic hyperinflation, breathlessness, and exercise performance during the 6-minute-walk test in chronic obstructive pulmonary disease. Am J Respir Crit Care Med. 2001;163:1395–9.
5. Elbehairy AF, Ciavaglia CE, Webb KA, Guenette JA, Jensen D, Mourad SM, et al. Pulmonary gas exchange abnormalities in mild chronic obstructive pulmonary disease. Implications for dyspnea and exercise intolerance. Am J Respir Crit Care Med. 2015;191(12):1384–94.
6. Bräunlich J, Köhler M, Wirtz H. Nasal high flow improves ventilation in patients with COPD. Int J Chron Obstruct Pulmon Dis. 2016;11:1077–85.
7. Möller W, Celik G, Feng S, Bartenstein P, Meyer G, Oliver E, et al. Nasal high flow clears anatomical dead space in upper airway models. J Appl Physiol (1985). 2015;118(12):1525–32.
8. Bräunlich J, Mauersberger F, Wirtz H. Effectiveness of nasal high flow in hypercapnic COPD patients is flow and leakage dependent. BMC Pulm Med. 2018;18:14.
9. O'Driscoll BR, Howard LS, Davison AG, British Thoracic Society. BTS guideline for emergency oxygen use in adult patients. Thorax. 2008;63(Suppl 6):vo1-68.
10. Spoletini G, Alotaibi M, Blasi F, Hill NS. Heated humidified high-flow nasal oxygen in adults: mechanisms of action and clinical implications. Chest. 2015;148:253–61.
11. Couser JI, Make BJ. Transtracheal oxygen decreases inspired minute ventilation. Am Rev Respir Dis. 1989;139:627–31.
12. Cirio S, Piran M, Vitacca M, Piaggi G, Ceriana P, Prazzoli M, et al. Effects of heated and humidified high flow gases during high-intensity constant-load exercise on severe COPD patients with ventilatory limitation. Respir Med. 2016;118:128–32.
13. Mündel T, Feng S, Tatkov S, Schneider H. Mechanisms of nasal high flow on ventilation during wakefulness and sleep. J Appl Physiol. 2013;114:1058–65.
14. Chanques G, Riboulet F, Molinari N, Carr J, Jung B, Prades A, et al. Comparison of three high flow oxygen therapy delivery devices: a clinical physiological cross-over study. Minerva Anestesiol. 2013;79:1344–55.
15. Kee K, Stuart-Andrews C, Ellis MJ. Increased dead space ventilation mediates reduced exercise capacity in systolic heart failure. Am J Respir Crit Care Med. 2016;193(11):1292–300.
16. Pitta F, Troosters T, Spruit MA, Probst VS, Dcramed M, Gosselink R. Characteristics of physical activities in daily life in chronic obstructive pulmonary disease. Am J Respir Crit Care Med. 2005;171:972–7.
17. Vaes AW, Garcia-Aymerich J, Marott JL, Benet M, Groenen MT, Schnohr P, et al. Changes in physical activity and all-cause mortality in COPD. Eur Respir J. 2014;44:1199–209.
18. Spruit MA, Pitta F, McAuley E, Zuwallack RL, Nici L. Pulmonary rehabilitation and physical activity in patients with chronic obstructive pulmonary disease. Am J Respir Crit Care Med. 2015;192:924–33.
19. Troosters T, Casaburi R, Gosselink R, Decramer M. Pulmonary rehabilitation in chronic obstructive pulmonary disease. Am J Respir Crit Care Med. 2005;172:19–38.
20. Dewan NA, Bell CW. Effect of low flow and high flow oxygen delivery on exercise tolerance and sensation of dyspnea. A study comparing the transtracheal catheter and nasal prongs. Chest. 1994;105:1061–5.
21. O'Donnell DE, D'Arsigny C, Webb K. Effects of hyperoxia on ventilatory limitation during exercise in advanced chronic obstructive pulmonary disease. Am J Respir Crit Care Med. 2001;163:892–8.
22. Nonoyama ML, Brooks D, Lacasse Y, Guyatt GH, Goldstein RS. Oxygen therapy during exercise training in chronic obstructive pulmonary disease. Cochrane Database Syst Rev. 2007;2:CD005372.
23. Jarosch I, Gloeckl R, Damm E, Schwedhelm AL, Buhrow D, Jerrentrup A, et al. Short-term effects of supplemental oxygen on 6-min walk test outcomes in patients with COPD: a randomized, placebo-controlled, single-blind, crossover trial. Chest. 2017;151(4):795–803.

24. Scanlan CL, Heuer A. Medical gas therapy. 8th ed. St Louis, MO: Egan's Fundamentals of Respiratory Care; 1999. p. 737–70.
25. Chatila W, Nugent T, Vance G, Gaughan J, Criner GJ. The effects of high-flow vs low-flow oxygen on exercise in advanced obstructive airways disease. Chest. 2004;126(4):1108–15.
26. Castellano Barneche MF, Dell'Era S, Roux N, Gimeno Santos E, Terrasa S, Bykhovsky I, et al. High flow nasal cannula improves exercise capacity in COPD patients: crossover trial. Eur Respir J. 201852:OA5196. https://doi.org/10.1183/13993003. Congress-2018. OA5196
27. Prieur G, Medrinal C, Combret Y, Quesada AR, Prieur F, Quieffin J, et al. Effect of high-flow nasal therapy during acute aerobic exercise in patients with chronic obstructive pulmonary disease after exacerbation: protocol for a randomised, controlled, cross-over trial. BMJ Open Respir Res. 2017;4(1):e000191.
28. Vitacca M, Paneroni M, Zampogna E, et al. High-flow oxygen therapy during exercise training in patients with chronic obstructive pulmonary disease and chronic hypoxemia: a multicenter randomized controlled trial. Phys Ther. 2020;100(8):1249–59. https://doi.org/10.1093/ptj/pzaa076.
29. Rossi V, Cirio S, Piran M, Bettinelli G, Zocchi L, Ceriana P, Carlucci A. High flow nasal cannula during walking in severe COPD patients: a randomized controlled trial. Eur Respir J. 201852:PA3645. https://doi.org/10.1183/13993003. Congress-2018. PA3645
30. Holland AE, Hill CJ, Conron M, Munro P, McDonald CF. Short term improvement in exercise capacity and symptoms following exercise training in interstitial lung disease. Thorax. 2008;63:549–54.
31. Nishiyama O, Kondoh Y, Kimura T, Kato K, Kataoka K, Ogawa T, et al. Effects of pulmonary rehabilitation in patients with idiopathic pulmonary fibrosis. Respirology. 2008;13:394–9.
32. King TE, Bradford WZ, Castro-Bernardini S, Fagan EA, Glaspole I, Glassberg MK, Gorina E, Hopkins PM, Kardatzke D, Lancaster L, et al. ASCEND study group. A phase 3 trial of pirfenidone in patients with idiopathic pulmonary fibrosis. N Engl J Med. 2014;370:2083–92.
33. Richeldi L, du Bois RM, Raghu G, Azuma A, Brown KK, Costabel U, Cottin V, Flaherty KR, Hansell DM, Inoue Y, INPULSIS Trial Investigators, et al. Efficacy and safety of nintedanib in idiopathic pulmonary fibrosis. N Engl J Med. 2014;370:2071–82.

Clinical Applications of High-Flow Nasal Cannula in Particular Settings: Invasive Procedures, Palliative Care and Transplantation

9

Umberto Lucangelo, Massimo Ferluga, Lucia Comuzzi, and Enrico Lena

9.1 Invasive Procedures

High-flow nasal cannulas (HFNC) are increasingly used in various clinical scenarios. Among them, there are some particular settings in which the device has started to be studied and applied in the last years. An interesting field of application of HFNC is invasive procedures, e.g., gastrointestinal endoscopies and bronchoscopy. Many invasive procedures are performed in non-operating room settings and under sedation. An important issue is the depth of sedation chosen for a particular procedure. In Table 9.1, the four stages of sedation are represented [1]: the decision to perform a procedure with no or some degree of sedation depends on the patient clinical conditions and/or the procedure itself, in addition to local habits.

The depth of sedation chosen helps also to define the type of monitoring required and the practitioner best involved to administer it: anaesthetists are trained to manage deep sedation and the airways, so they should be involved in more complex cases. A combination of sedative and analgesic medication may be administered as appropriate.

During sedation, it is recommended to monitor the level of consciousness; the ventilatory function by observation of the patient, capnography (if possible) and pulse oximetry; and the haemodynamics through blood pressure, heart rate and electrocardiographic monitoring [2].

A common adverse event during sedation is hypoxaemia, which is related to respiratory depression caused by sedative/analgesic drugs, airway obstruction and decreased compliance of the chest wall [3]. Hypoxaemia can cause complications like myocardial ischaemia, arrhythmias, neurological damage and death [4–6].

U. Lucangelo (✉) · M. Ferluga · L. Comuzzi · E. Lena
Emergency and Urgency Department, Azienda Sanitaria Universitaria Giuliano Isontina, Trieste, Italy
e-mail: u.lucangelo@fmc.units.it

© Springer Nature Switzerland AG 2021
A. Carlucci, S. M. Maggiore (eds.), *High Flow Nasal Cannula*,
https://doi.org/10.1007/978-3-030-42454-1_9

Table 9.1 Stages of sedation

Clinical effect	Minimal sedation	Moderate sedation	Deep sedation	General anaesthesia
Responsiveness	To verbal stimulation	Purposeful response to verbal or tactile stimulation	Purposeful response after repeated and/or painful stimulation	Unresponsive to verbal/tactile or painful stimulation
Airway control	Not affected	Minimal effect	May need intervention	Always need intervention
Ventilation	Spontaneous	Spontaneous	May need assistance	Always need assistance, albeit spontaneous ventilation can be achieved
Haemodynamic stability	Not affected	Minimal effect	Minimal effect	Always affected, may require intervention

Another important issue is that in some cases, for technical reasons, the practitioner who is performing the procedure and the anaesthetist have to share the airways, making their management more challenging. For these reasons, it is recommended to administer supplemental oxygen for moderate and deeper stages of sedation [2].

In this context, HFNC seems to be a useful tool to administer oxygen during sedation, because of its effect on maintaining a stable fraction of inspired oxygen (FiO_2), its potential for apnoeic oxygenation and carbon dioxide (CO_2) washout.

9.2 Gastrointestinal Endoscopies

Gastrointestinal endoscopies vary wildly based on the type and complexity of the procedure. A case series and only one study have described the use of HFNC during colonoscopy in obese patients [7–8]. This is probably the simplest procedure regarding airway and oxygenation management as the airway is not shared. However, obese population frequently present difficult airway and ventilation management, so HFNC may be a useful device to be applied in such patients. Riccio et al. performed a randomized control trial (RCT) to compare HFNC with standard nasal cannulas during colonoscopy in 59 morbidly obese patients under deep sedation. They found no difference regarding the number of desaturation episodes between the groups. However, in the subgroup with a high probability of obstructive sleep apnoea, HFNC seemed to perform better than standard nasal cannulas, indicating a possible role of the device in this population [8].

Lin et al. compared HFNC with standard nasal cannula in almost 2000 low-risk patients during gastroscopy, finding that HFNC decreases the incidence of hypoxaemia [9].

Endoscopic retrograde cholangiopancreatography (ERCP) is a challenging procedure because it frequently takes a long time and requires deep sedation, the airways are not easily accessible and the patient is often prone. A retrospective study examined the role of HFNC during ERCP and endoscopic ultrasound and found that the use of the device was associated with improved oxygenation when compared with standard nasal cannulas, in addition to a decreased use of general anaesthesia [10].

As evident, only few studies have been performed on this topic. We can conclude that HFNC seems to be a useful tool in some cases but future research is needed to assess which procedures and/or patients would benefit most from its application.

9.3   Bronchoscopy

Bronchoscopy is a challenging procedure regarding the management of oxygenation and ventilation, because it requires the airway to be partially obstructed by instrumentation and can lead itself to desaturation. Moreover, it can be associated with diagnostic and/or therapeutic interventions that may compromise oxygenation and ventilation further.

Many studies have been conducted on the use of HFNC to support the ventilatory function during this procedure.

The first study that examined HFNC during flexible bronchoscopy with bronchoalveolar lavage (BAL) was conducted on non-hypoxaemic mildly sedated patients by our group. We found that HFNC with a flow of 60 L/min performed better than a flow of 40 L/min and Venturi mask in terms of oxygenation during the procedure and return to baseline arterial CO_2 level after the procedure. It must be pointed out, however, that no episodes of desaturation were detected in any group. Moreover, we demonstrated in healthy volunteers that a flow of 60 L/min was able to generate a small positive end-expiratory airway pressure (PEEP) even with the mouth open, while a flow of 40 L/min could not [11].

In another study, HFNC at a flow of 30–70 L/min was compared with standard nasal cannula at 10–15 L/min during endobronchial ultrasound (EBUS) and a better oxygenation was demonstrated with the former. However, the number of episodes of desaturation during the procedure did not differ between groups, highlighting that HFNC does not completely protect against this complication [12].

Later, the attention of other authors started to focus on hypoxaemic patients. Observational studies found HFNC to perform good during bronchoscopy in these patients [13–15]. Moreover, two RCT have been published on this topic. It is known that non-invasive ventilation (NIV) can prevent desaturation during bronchoscopy better than conventional oxygen delivery [16–23]. Simon et al. [24] compared the use of HFNC with a flow of 50 L/min versus NIV during bronchoscopy in 40 critically ill patients with acute hypoxemic respiratory failure, which are well known to be more prone to develop procedure-related complications [25]. They demonstrated that NIV was associated with better oxygenation before, during and after the procedure. However, the lowest peripheral oxygen saturation (SpO_2) during bronchoscopy did not differ between groups, and no $SpO_2 < 85\%$ was recorded in any group. Indeed, the authors concluded that NIV is superior to HFNC in this context;

however, in patients stable on HFNC before the procedure, it can be well tolerated with this device [24].

Another study by Saksitthichok et al. compared HFNC at a lower flow (40 L/min) with NIV during diagnostic bronchoscopy for pulmonary lesions in 51 hypoxemic patients. SpO_2 was maintained at acceptable levels in both groups; however, the lowest $SpO_2 < 90\%$ tended to occur more often with HFNC. Moreover, NIV was associated with better oxygenation in patients who presented a worse baseline oxygenation and a better stability of oxygenation and ventilatory and haemodynamics parameters [26].

These results can be explained by the fact that with the mouth open the flow delivered with HFNC may be insufficient to generate a PEEP effect, as depicted by Lucangelo et al. [11], and to guarantee a constant FiO_2, as can be hypothesized that a patient with respiratory failure during bronchoscopy may present a peak inspiratory flow rate higher than that used with HFNC in the two studies.

These results indicate that HFNC may be a valid alternative to NIV in mild/moderate hypoxaemic patients, but NIV performs better in terms of oxygenation in all patients and is necessary in severe cases. However, more studies are needed to assess this hypothesis and to test higher flows with HFNC.

In relation to rigid bronchoscopy, there is only a case series which describes the use of HFNC for preoxygenation with good results. However, the patients were ventilated during the procedure. Indeed, there is no report on the use of the device to maintain apnoeic oxygenation throughout it, although other studies and reports have described this use during airway surgery [27–34].

9.4   Other Procedures

A case report describes the successful use of HFNC in a patient with respiratory failure who underwent percutaneous balloon aortic valvuloplasty under transoesophageal echocardiographic monitoring [35].

In conclusion, even if at the present time the evidence regarding the use of the device in invasive procedure is not robust, HFNC may be effective in many scenarios. More studies are needed to assess which procedures and especially which patients will benefit most from its use.

9.5   Palliative Care

The goals of palliative care defined by the World Health Organization are the improvement of the quality of life of patients and their families facing the problems associated with life-threatening illness. This approach involves prevention and relief of suffering by means of early identification and impeccable assessment and treatment of pain and other problems (physical, psychosocial and spiritual) [36]. One of the major objectives of palliative care is the relief of dyspnoea. It has been reported that the majority of patients affected by chronic obstructive pulmonary disease (COPD), heart failure or cancer experience dyspnoea near the end of their life [37].

Supplemental oxygen is frequently prescribed to reduce shortness of breath even when patients are not hypoxemic [38]. However recent guidelines do not support with a strong level of evidence the use of oxygen as a relief for non-hypoxaemic patients [39]. On the other hand, there is a consistent number of studies demonstrating the futility of oxygen supplementation to treat breathing discomfort. In fact, there seem to be no differences between delivering room air and oxygen with a facial mask [40]. Interestingly a relevant degree of comfort can be provided by placing a fan in front of a patient's face [40, 41]. The physical stimulation of nasal and oral mucosa may decrease breathlessness.

Another device frequently used in palliative care is NIV, which is considered a cornerstone in the management of COPD exacerbations, cardiogenic pulmonary oedema and in general in immunosuppressed patients with respiratory failure [42, 43].

However, despite the advantages in terms of symptom relief and short-term survival, this kind of respiratory support has been seen as unnecessary or even harmful in a palliative care scenario.

The first study was published in 1994 by Meduri and investigated the use of NIV in a cohort of patients with respiratory failure refusing intubation. They concluded that mechanical ventilation via oronasal face mask provided an effective, comfortable and dignified method of supporting patients in that clinical setting [44]. From that time on several clinical studies had been investigating this topic finding that NIV can improve the quality of life and alleviate dyspnoea. In addition, if patients with COPD or cardiogenic dyspnoea were treated with NIV, survival and hospital discharge improved even in the presence of a not-to-intubate order [45–48]. These results were confirmed by Wilson in a recent meta-analysis that included 33 studies. The authors found that a significant proportion of subjects with do-not-intubate orders survived to hospital discharge (56%) and at 1 year (32%). Survival was better for subjects with COPD (68% to hospital discharge) and cardiopulmonary oedema (68% to hospital discharge) but worse for subjects with pneumonia (41% to hospital discharge) and malignancy (37% to hospital discharge) [49]. The European Respiratory Society and the American Thoracic Society published in 2017 the clinical practice guidelines for the use of NIV in acute respiratory failure. In the section regarding palliative care the authors refer to three different clinical settings described in a past article [50]: type 1 scenario consists of life support without limits, type 2 life support with preset limits (do-not-intubate) and type 3 just comfort measures. The main difference between type 2 and type 3 is that in type 2 the ventilatory support is prescribed while the underlying cause of the respiratory failure is being treated and therefore the patient can improve and even be discharged. For this reason, a certain degree of discomfort could be tolerated as long as the treatment is effective. The guidelines state that, due to the lack of RCT evidence, no recommendation can be made for type 2 patients. However, the authors underlined that, in observational studies, the use of NIV in "do-not-intubate" patients was associated, at least in some subsets of patients (COPD and congestive heart failure), with a surprisingly high (>30–60%) hospital survival and a 3-month quality of life equivalent to patients treated with NIV and having no limitation placed on support. On the other hand, the guidelines recommend with a moderate certainty of evidence the use of NIV in the type 3 scenario if it improves breathlessness and respiratory distress without causing other troubling consequences, such as mask discomfort or unduly prolonging life [51]. Therefore, if the breathing mask is not well tolerated or the patient cannot communicate satisfactorily or the dyspnoea does not improve, the treatment has to be interrupted.

HFNC is another kind of respiratory support that delivers heated and humidified oxygen at high flow rates [52]. Compared to other devices, HFNC provides a number of physiological benefits including greater comfort and tolerance, more effective oxygenation under some circumstances and breathing pattern improvements with an increase in tidal volume and decreases in respiratory rate and dyspnoea. These benefits are broadening the indications of HFNC, which has now been evaluated and used to treat hypoxaemic respiratory failure, to improve oxygenation for pre-intubation, and to treat patients after surgery or after extubation [53].

However just a few clinical studies have addressed the use of HFNC in the palliative care and more in detail in patients with do-not-intubate order. In 2013 Peters et al. [54] published a retrospective analysis of 50 patients with do-not-intubate status treated with high-flow nasal cannula for respiratory failure. The aim of the study was to investigate the effectiveness of HFNC in terms of patient tolerance, change in respiratory variables and need for NIV. Fifty patients admitted during a 2-year period in the Mayo Clinic in Rochester, Minnesota, were included with the following criteria: do-not-intubate or resuscitate status, evidence of respiratory distress (dyspnoea, tachypnoea), hypoxaemia and mild or compensated hypercapnia. Patients were excluded if there was no intention to escalate to NIV which means that the role of HFNC in the aforementioned type 3 clinical setting was not taken into consideration. Therapy was initiated at previous FiO_2 and a flow of 35 L/min, titrating flow upward if tolerated to 45–50 L/ min. FiO_2 was then titrated to maintain SaO_2 at 90%, or according to specific clinical orders. Mean age was 73 years and the diagnoses were quite different with two-thirds of the patient affected by a respiratory pathology (pulmonary fibrosis, pneumonia and COPD). Before treatment patients presented with a mild hypoxia (mean PaO_2 of 66.5 mmHg) and a normal acid-base status (mean pH of 7.42). Data regarding post-treatment blood gas analysis are lacking and no statistical analysis was reported. However other respiratory variables such as mean oxygen saturation and breathing frequency were considered. HFNC treatment induced a general improvement with a significant increase in mean oxygen saturation (from 89.1% to 94.7%) and significant reduction of the breathing frequency (from 30.6 breaths/min to 24.7 breaths/min). Nine patients (18%) escalated to NIV and six of them (67%) died while the mortality in the group treated only with HFNC was 58% (p 0.72). In line with the present literature a better outcome was observed for the patients with a reversible cause of respiratory failure such as congestive heart failure or acute exacerbation of COPD [55]. Median duration of use of HFNC was 30 h and the treatment was well tolerated, with no episodes of nasal bleeding or facial skin breakdown. In spite of the limitations (like the sample size, the miscellaneous diagnosis and the lack of data) some interesting conclusions can be drawn. Firstly, HFNC can be tolerated for a consistent amount of time without causing discomfort of facial lesions. Secondly this treatment can improve some respiratory variables with a decreased need for NIV. Thirdly, since HFNC requires less training than NIV, these patients could be efficiently treated outside the ICU environment even if this hypothesis is not tested in the present study.

Similar results can be found in a retrospective analysis published by Epstein in 2011 comprehending 183 cancer-affected patients (including 101 with do-not-resuscitate orders) treated with HFNC [56]. Almost the whole population had some degree of hypoxia and the majority (72%) was admitted in an ICU. In general, the device was well tolerated with just two patients reporting nasal discomfort and the median time of treatment was 3 days. HFNC was effective in the management of respiratory difficulties: 41% of patients improved whereas 44% remained stable and only 15% declined. It is worth noting that 13 patients were taken care of in the ward avoiding the ICU admission. This study, even if it does not provide information with a high level of evidence, shows that HFNC is well tolerated among a cancer-affected population. Moreover, this treatment can help patients deal with respiratory difficulties and decrease the need for other kinds of ventilatory support. However, it has to be pointed out that the sample size comprehended patients with both "do-not-intubate" and "full-code" status.

In 2013 David Hui addressed the effect on dyspnoea of two different kinds of respiratory support designing a phase two randomized trial [57]. Thirty patients were included in the study with the following criteria: diagnosis of advanced cancer, presence of dyspnoea (at least 3/10 on a numeric rating scale) despite supplemental oxygen, no neurological impairment and life expectancy of more than 1 week. The patients were then randomly assigned to receive 2 h of HFNC followed by a variable washout period and then 2 h of BiPAP or 2 h of BiPAP followed by a variable washout period and then 2 h of HFNC. However, several patients were not able to complete both steps so only the first phase was considered and the study was analysed as a parallel study. All interventions were delivered in acute care units outside of the intensive care setting, the average level of oxygen flow on HFNC was 21 L/min while the average BiPAP inspiratory pressure was 9 cmH$_2$O and expiratory pressure was set at 5 cmH$_2$O. A total of 23 patients were included: 13 treated with HFNC and 10 treated with BiPAP. The intensity of dyspnoea was examined using both the NRS and the modified Borg scale (MBS). Both the treatments were associated with an average dyspnoea improvement. No significant differences in dyspnoea relief were detected between the two devices. Moreover, BiPAP was associated with a decrease in heart rate while a significant decrease in systolic blood pressure and a rise in oxygen saturation were observed in the HFNC group. No adverse effects with BiPAP or HFNC were described but patients reported less trouble sleeping while on HFO as compared with BiPAP. Interestingly, this study suggests that HFNC can be as effective as NIV in relieving from dyspnoea with better tolerance especially during night-time. Furthermore, it has to be pointed out that a reduction of dyspnoea does not necessarily imply an increment of oxygen saturation and these data are in line with this statement.

A recent paper published by Koyauchi et al. in 2018 focused on the efficacy and tolerability of HFNC in terminal patients affected by interstitial lung fibrosis [58]. This was a retrospective single-centre study that included patients matching the criteria listed below: diagnosis of interstitial lung fibrosis, acute hypoxemic respiratory failure treated with either HFNC or NIV and do-not-intubate status. Therefore, the included patients were divided into two groups in consideration of the treatment received (HFNC or NIV). The outcome measures were 30-day survival, in-hospital mortality, temporary interruption at the patient's request, discontinuation at the patient's request, respiratory rate, dyspnoea, and the patient's ability to eat and to converse with family or caregivers at the end of life. Fifty-four patients were treated with HFNC for a median of 7 days and a median flow rate of 40 L/min while NIV was administered to 30 patients for a median time of 5 days. No differences were observed between these two groups in terms of hospital mortality and 30-day survival, but both the temporary interruption rates and discontinuation rates were lower among patients treated with HFNC. Similarly, these patients were significantly better able to eat and to converse before death and experienced fewer adverse events in comparison to the NIV group. Dyspnoea scores did not change significantly between pre- and post-treatment in either group, but respiratory rate decreased significantly after the therapy with HFNC.

In conclusion the present literature suggests that HFNC can be useful in the palliative care settings because they are well tolerated, even for a consistent period of time, with few adverse events and they can be managed outside the ICU. Moreover, this treatment could mitigate dyspnoea and improve some respiratory variables while patients are able to eat and communicate with their relatives. However, these statements cannot be supported by a strong level of evidence due to the limitations of the aforementioned studies.

In closing, Davies in 2019 [55] summarized a series of questions that have to be answered by patients, families and clinicians before choosing any kind of ventilatory support at the end of life: How long will it prolong life? Will it restore or maintain alertness? Will the therapy increase or relieve suffering?

9.6 Transplantation

The populations of living immunocompromised patients have been increasing in the last decade and include active cancer, organ transplant, use of immunosuppressive agents and chemotherapy; new treatments in autoimmune conditions and solid organ transplantation and greater life expectancy in cancer patients are the main determinants of this improvement [59]. Nevertheless, immunocompromised patients also carry higher risks of many life-threatening complications and, among these, acute respiratory failure (ARF) is the leading cause of intensive care unit (ICU) admission [60]. Once these patients evolve into ARF, they often need endotracheal intubation and invasive mechanical ventilation (IMV), both associated with an increase in morbidity and mortality, due to the risk of bacterial, viral or opportunistic infections [61]. Several studies have shown that NIV is associated with decreased mortality in immunocompromised patients; however, a multicentre, randomized clinical study just showed that NIV did not provide an additional survival benefit compared with standard oxygen therapy [62]. Nevertheless, NIV is still recommended a first-line strategy for immunocompromised patients with ARF.

HFNC represents a valid alternative to NIV in patients with ARF and its use in immunocompromised patients was described in small and single-centre studies, or post hoc analyses in limited number of patients provided conflicting information [63, 64].

The Efraim multinational prospective cohort study evaluated in 1611 immuno-compromised patients the effects of initial ventilatory strategies on intubation, mechanical ventilation and hospital mortality; as already seen in immunocompetent patients, HFNC reduced intubation rate but did not influence hospital mortality. More interesting was the association between the causes of ARF and outcomes: patients with unknown cause were at high risk of death. This could be due to the wrong choice of oxygenation device that could cause delay of an appropriate diagnostic workup and failure to recognize and treat a pulmonary complication [60].

Recently, systematic reviews and meta-analysis compared HFNC with other respiratory support techniques in immunocompromised patients with ARF and its effect in terms of reduction of short-term mortality, intubation rate and ICU length of stay. In 2015 Lee and colleagues investigated the feasibility of HFNC use in 45 patients with haematologic malignancies and ARF. Interestingly, the percentage of bacterial pneumonia was significantly higher in the HFNC treatment failure group compared with the success group (73.3% vs. 26.7%; $P = 0.004$), but the aetiology of respiratory failure has not been found to be associated with the success of HFNC therapy. More than 30% of the patients studied successfully recovered from ARF without the use of mechanical ventilation and the author stressed the importance of establishing criteria for the selection of an HFNC as the initial ventilator therapy [65].

HFNC was successfully used in 37 lung transplant recipients readmitted to the ICU because of ARF; as could be expected, patients who succeeded on HFNC had better outcomes in survival and ICU length of stay compared with patients who failed, and, more importantly, no adverse effects during HFNC were observed. Other advantages of the use of nasal cannulas were the possibility of nasogastric tube feeding, phonation, chest physiotherapy and coughing. Moreover, the authors observed that maintaining an adequate oxygenation, decreasing respiratory rate and consequently avoiding organ failure were the most significant determinants of HFNC treatment success [66]. In 38 renal transplant recipients with ARF secondary to severe pneumonia Tu and colleagues demonstrated in 2017 that HFNC therapy achieved the same outcomes of NIV, but the total number of ventilator-free days at day 28 was significantly higher in the HFNC group, where a significant lower incidence of pneumothorax and skin breakdown was observed. In this study, two important issues should be highlighted: first, the patients in the HFNC group, which received NIV as salvage treatment and then underwent salvage intubation, had a worse outcome, due to the delayed intubation; second, the ICU and in-hospital mortality was not influenced by the type of the initial ventilator support, but by the severity of illness [67].

Gaspari and colleagues conducted the first clinical study that explored the usefulness of the preventive application of HFNC after elective extubation in 29 patients undergoing liver transplantation; the latter usually have several concomitant morbidities that increase the risk of postextubation hypoxemia and postoperative pulmonary complications. Surprisingly, when compared with subjects who were critically ill with ARF, the routine use of HFNC did not reduce the incidence of hypoxaemia, weaning failure, ICU length of stay or 28-day mortality. The authors remarked the simplicity of use of HFNC, particularly for their tolerance and comfort; moreover, the use of a high-flow system was economical because it was integrated into the ICU ventilator [68].

In conclusion, the use of HFNC may reduce the need of intubation and mechanical ventilation in immunocompromised patients with ARF, but there is not enough evidence to support its widespread use. Further large, high-quality, randomized, multicentre trials are needed to confirm the effects of HFNC on survival and LOS in the ICU or in hospital.

References

1. American Society of Anesthesiologists. Continuum of Depth of Sedation: Definition of General Anesthesia and Levels of Sedation/Analgesia. Last amended on October 17, 2018.
2. Practice guidelines for moderate procedural sedation and analgesia 2018: a report by the American Society of Anesthesiologists Task Force on Moderate Procedural Sedation and Analgesia, the American Association of Oral and Maxillofacial Surgeons, American College of Radiology, American Dental Association, American Society of Dentist Anesthesiologists, and Society of Interventional Radiology. Anesthesiology. 2018;128:437–79.
3. Amornyotin S. Sedation-related complications in gastrointestinal endoscopy. World J Gastrointest Endosc. 2013;5:527–33.
4. Qadeer MA, Lopez AR, Dumot JA, et al. Hypoxemia during moderate sedation for gastrointestinal endoscopy: causes and associations. Digestion. 2011;84:37–45.
5. Xiao Q, Yang Y, Zhou Y, et al. Comparison of nasopharyngeal airway device and nasal oxygen tube in obese patients undergoing intravenous anesthesia for gastroscopy: a prospective and randomized study. Gastroenterol Res Pract. 2016;2016:2641257.
6. Patterson KW, Noonan N, Keeling NW. Hypoxemia during outpatient gastrointestinal endoscopy: the effects of sedation and supplemental oxygen. J Clin Anesth. 1995;7:136–40.
7. Lee CC, Perez O, Farooqi FI, et al. Use of high-flow nasal cannula in obese patients receiving colonoscopy under intravenous propofol sedation: a case series. Respir Med Case Rep. 2018;23:118–21.
8. Riccio CA, Sarmiento S, Minhajuddin A, et al. High-flow versus standard nasal cannula in morbidly obese patients during colonoscopy: a prospective, randomized clinical trial. J Clin Anesth. 2019;54:19–24.
9. Lin Y, Zhang X, Li L, et al. High-flow nasal cannula oxygen therapy and hypoxia during gastroscopy with propofol sedation: a randomized multicenter clinical trial. Gastrointest Endosc. 2019;90:591–601.

10. Schumann R, Natov NS, Rocuts-Martinez KA, et al. High-flow nasal oxygen availability for sedation decreases the use of general anesthesia during endoscopic retrograde cholangiopancreatography and endoscopic ultrasound. World J Gastroenterol. 2016;22:10398–405.
11. Lucangelo U, Vassallo FG, Marras E, et al. High-flow nasal interface improves oxygenation in patients undergoing bronchoscopy. Crit Care Res Pract. 2012;2012:506382.
12. Douglas N, Ng I, Nazeem F, et al. A randomised controlled trial comparing high-flow nasal oxygen with standard management for conscious sedation during bronchoscopy. Anaesthesia. 2018;73:169–76.
13. Chung SM, Choi JW, Lee YS, et al. Clinical effectiveness of high-flow nasal cannula in hypoxaemic patients during bronchoscopic procedures. Tuberc Respir Dis. 2019;82:81–5.
14. Kim EJ, Jung CY, Kim KC. Effectiveness and safety of high-flow nasal cannula oxygen delivery during bronchoalveolar lavage in acute respiratory failure patients. Tuberc Respir Dis. 2018;81:319–29.
15. La Combe B, Messika J, Labbé V, et al. High-flow nasal oxygen for bronchoalveolar lavage in acute respiratory failure patients. Eur Respir J. 2016;47:1283–6.
16. Antonelli M, Conti G, Riccioni L, et al. Noninvasive positive-pressure ventilation via face mask during bronchoscopy with BAL in high-risk hypoxemic patients. Chest. 1996;110:724–8.
17. Da Conceiçao M, Genco G, Favier JC, et al. Fiber-optic bronchoscopy during noninvasive positive-pressure ventilation in patients with chronic obstructive lung disease with hypoxemia and hypercapnia. Ann Fr Anesth Reanim. 2000;19:231–6.
18. Maitre B, Jaber S, Maggiore SM, et al. Continuous positive airway pressure during fiber-optic bronchoscopy in hypoxemic patients. A randomized double-blind study using a new device. Am J Respir Crit Care Med. 2000;162:1063–7.
19. Antonelli M, Conti G, Rocco M, et al. Noninvasive positive-pressure ventilation vs. conventional oxygen supplementation in hypoxemic patients undergoing diagnostic bronchoscopy. Chest. 2002;121:1149–54.
20. Antonelli M, Pennisi MA, Conti G, et al. Fiberoptic bronchoscopy during noninvasive positive pressure ventilation delivered by helmet. Intensive Care Med. 2003;29:126–9.
21. Chiner E, Llombart M, Signes-Costa J, et al. Description of a new procedure for fiber-optic bronchoscopy during noninvasive ventilation through a nasal mask in patients with acute respiratory failure. Arch Bronconeumol. 2005;41:698–701.
22. Heunks LM, de Bruin CJ, van der Hoeven JG, et al. Non-invasive mechanical ventilation for diagnostic bronchoscopy using a new face mask: an observational feasibility study. Intensive Care Med. 2010;36:143–7.
23. Cracco C, Fartoukh M, Prodanovic H, et al. Safety of performing fiber-optic bronchoscopy in critically ill hypoxemic patients with acute respiratory failure. Intensive Care Med. 2013;39:45–52.
24. Simon M, Braune S, Frings D, et al. High-flow nasal cannula oxygen versus non-invasive ventilation in patients with acute hypoxaemic respiratory failure undergoing flexible bronchoscopy—a prospective randomised trial. Crit Care. 2014;18:712.
25. Albertini RE, Harrell JH 2nd, Kurihara N, et al. Arterial hypoxemia induced by fiber-optic bronchoscopy. JAMA. 1974;230:1666–7.
26. Saksitthichok B, Petnak T, So-Ngern A, et al. A prospective randomized comparative study of high-flow nasal cannula oxygen and non-invasive ventilation in hypoxemic patients undergoing diagnostic flexible bronchoscopy. J Thorac Dis. 2019;11:1929–39.
27. Bourn S, Milligan P, McNarry AF. Use of transnasal humidified rapid-insufflation ventilatory exchange (THRIVE) to facilitate the management of subglottic stenosis in pregnancy. Int J Obstet Anesth. 2019;19. [Epub ahead of print]
28. Damrose EJ, Manson L, Nekhendzy V, et al. Management of subglottic stenosis in pregnancy using advanced apnoeic ventilatory techniques. J Laryngol Otol. 2019;133:399–403.
29. Desai N, Fowler A. Use of Transnasal humidified rapid-insufflation ventilatory exchange for emergent surgical tracheostomy: a case report. A A Case Rep. 2017;9:268–70.
30. Ebeling CG, Riccio CA. Apneic oxygenation with high-flow nasal cannula and transcutaneous carbon dioxide monitoring during airway surgery: a case series. A A Pract. 2019;12:366–8.

31. Fung R, Stellios J, Bannon PG, et al. Elective use of veno-venous extracorporeal membrane oxygenation and high-flow nasal oxygen for resection of subtotal malignant distal airway obstruction. Anaesth Intensive Care. 2017;45:88–91.
32. Lyons C, Callaghan M. Apnoeic oxygenation with high-flow nasal oxygen for laryngeal surgery: a case series. Anaesthesia. 2017;72:1379–87.
33. Patel A, Nouraei SA. Transnasal humidified rapid-insufflation ventilatory exchange (THRIVE): a physiological method of increasing apnoea time in patients with difficult airways. Anaesthesia. 2015;70:323–9.
34. Tam K, Jeffery C, Sung CK. Surgical management of supraglottic stenosis using intubationless optiflow. Ann Otol Rhinol Laryngol. 2017;126:669–72.
35. Sakazaki R, Suzuki T, Ikeda N. High-flow nasal cannula oxygen supported-transesophageal echocardiography under sedation in a respiratory compromised patient. J Cardiothorac Vasc Anesth. 2019;33:255–6.
36. World Health Association Palliative Care Fact Sheet.
37. Lynn J, Teno JM, Phillips RS, et al. Perceptions by family members of the dying experience of older and seriously ill patients. SUPPORT Investigators. Study to understand prognoses and preferences for outcomes and risks of treatments. Ann Intern Med. 1997;126:97–106.
38. Booth S, Wade R, Johnson M, et al. The use of oxygen in the palliation of breathlessness. A report of the expert working group of the scientific committee of the association of palliative medicine. Respir Med. 2004;98:66–77.
39. Lanken PN, Terry PB, Delisser HM, et al. An official American Thoracic Society clinical policy statement: palliative care for patients with respiratory diseases and critical illnesses. Am J Respir Crit Care Med. 2008;177:912–27.
40. Abernethy AP, McDonald CF, Frith PA, et al. Effect of palliative oxygen versus room air in relief of breathlessness in patients with refractory dyspnoea: a double-blind, randomised controlled trial. Lancet. 2010;376:784–93.
41. Galbraith S, Fagan P, Perkins P, et al. Does the use of a handheld fan improve chronic dyspnea? A randomized, controlled, crossover trial. J Pain Symptom Manag. 2010;39:831–8.
42. Lightowler JV, Wedzicha JA, Elliott MW, et al. Non-invasive positive pressure ventilation to treat respiratory failure resulting from exacerbations of chronic obstructive pulmonary disease: Cochrane systematic review and meta-analysis. BMJ. 2003;326:185.
43. Masip J, Roque M, Sánchez B, et al. Noninvasive ventilation in acute cardiogenic pulmonary edema: systematic review and meta-analysis. JAMA. 2005;294:3124–30.
44. Meduri GU, Fox RC, Abou-Shala N, et al. Noninvasive mechanical ventilation via face mask in patients with acute respiratory failure who refused endotracheal intubation. Crit Care Med. 1994;22:1584–90.
45. Levy M, Tanios MA, Nelson D, et al. Outcomes of patients with do-not-intubate orders treated with noninvasive ventilation. Crit Care Med. 2004;32:2002–7.
46. Schettino G, Altobelli N, Kacmarek RM. Noninvasive positive pressure ventilation reverses acute respiratory failure in select "do-not-intubate" patients. Crit Care Med. 2005;33:1976–82.
47. Meert AP, Berghmans T, Hardy M, et al. Non-invasive ventilation for cancer patients with life-support techniques limitation. Support Care Cancer. 2006;14:167–71.
48. Fernandez R, Baigorri F, Artigas A. Noninvasive ventilation in patients with "do-not-intubate" orders: medium-term efficacy depends critically on patient selection. Intensive Care Med. 2007;33:350–4.
49. Wilson ME, Majzoub AM, Dobler CC, et al. Noninvasive ventilation in patients with do-not-intubate and comfort-measures-only orders: a systematic review and meta-analysis. Crit Care Med. 2018;46:1209–16.
50. Curtis JR, Cook DJ, Sinuff T, et al. Noninvasive positive pressure ventilation in critical and palliative care settings: understanding the goals of therapy. Crit Care Med. 2007;35:932–9.
51. Rochwerg B, Brochard L, Elliott MW, et al. Official ERS/ATS clinical practice guidelines: noninvasive ventilation for acute respiratory failure. Eur Respir J. 2017;50
52. Spoletini G, Alotaibi M, Blasi F, et al. Heated humidified high-flow nasal oxygen in adults: mechanisms of action and clinical implications. Chest. 2015;148:253–61.

53. Azoulay E, Lemiale V, Mokart D, et al. High-flow nasal oxygen vs. standard oxygen therapy in immunocompromised patients with acute respiratory failure: study protocol for a randomized controlled trial. Trials. 2018;19:157.
54. Peters SG, Holets SR, Gay PC. High-flow nasal cannula therapy in do-not-intubate patients with hypoxemic respiratory distress. Respir Care. 2013;58:597–600.
55. Davies JD. Noninvasive respiratory support at the end of life. Respir Care. 2019;64:701–11.
56. Epstein AS, Hartridge-Lambert SK, Ramaker JS, et al. Humidified high-flow nasal oxygen utilization in patients with cancer at Memorial Sloan-Kettering Cancer Center. J Palliat Med. 2011;14:835–9.
57. Hui D, Morgado M, Chisholm G, et al. High-flow oxygen and bilevel positive airway pressure for persistent dyspnea in patients with advanced cancer: a phase II randomized trial. J Pain Symptom Manag. 2013;46:463–73.
58. Koyauchi T, Hasegawa H, Kanata K, et al. Efficacy and tolerability of high-flow nasal cannula oxygen therapy for hypoxemic respiratory failure in patients with interstitial lung disease with do-not-intubate orders: a retrospective single-center study. Respiration. 2018;96:323–9.
59. Allemani C, Weir HK, Carreira H, et al. Global surveillance of cancer survival 1995–2009: analysis of individual data for 25 676 887 patients from 279 population-based registries in 67 countries (CONCORD-2). Lancet. 2015;385:977–1010.
60. Azoulay E, Pickkers P, Soares M, et al. Acute hypoxemic respiratory failure in immunocompromised patients: the Efraim multinational prospective cohort study. Intensive Care Med. 2017;43:1808–19.
61. Moreau AS, Martin-Loeches I, et al. Impact of immunosuppression on incidence, aetiology and outcome of ventilator-associated lower respiratory tract infections. Eur Respir J. 2018;51:1701656.
62. Lemiale V, Mokart D, Resche-Rigon M, et al. Effect of noninvasive ventilation vs oxygen therapy on mortality among immunocompromised patients with acute respiratory failure: a randomized clinical trial. JAMA. 2015;314:1711–9.
63. Ou X, Hua Y, Liu J, et al. Effect of high-flow nasal cannula oxygen therapy in adults with acute hypoxemic respiratory failure: a meta-analysis of randomized controlled trials. Can Med Assoc J. 2017;189:E260–7.
64. Ni YN, Luo J, Yu H, et al. The effect of high-flow nasal cannula in reducing the mortality and the rate of endotracheal intubation when used before mechanical ventilation compared with conventional oxygen therapy and noninvasive positive pressure ventilation. A systematic review and meta-analysis. Am J Emerg Med. 2018;36:226–33.
65. Lee HY, Rhee CK, Lee JW. Feasibility of high-flow nasal cannula oxygen therapy for acute respiratory failure in patients with hematologic malignancies: a retrospective single-center study. J Crit Care. 2015;30:773–7.
66. Roca O, de Acilu MG, Caralt B, et al. Humidified high flow nasal cannula supportive therapy improves outcomes in lung transplant recipients readmitted to the intensive care unit because of acute respiratory failure. Transplantation. 2015;99:1092–8.
67. Tu G, He H, Yin K, et al. High-flow nasal cannula versus noninvasive ventilation for treatment of acute hypoxemic respiratory failure in renal transplant recipients. Transplant Proc. 2017;49:1325–30.
68. Gaspari R, Spinazzola G, Ferrone G, et al. High-flow nasal cannula versus standard oxygen therapy after extubation in liver transplantation: a matched controlled study. Respir Care. 2020;65:21–8.

Physiological Effects and Clinical Applications of High-Flow Nasal Cannula in Children

10

Giovanna Chidini and Edoardo Calderini

10.1 Introduction

In pediatric age, acute respiratory failure [ARF] represents one of the main causes for hospitalization in developed and incoming countries with a pediatric intensive care unit [PICU] admission rate ranging from 2% to 6% [1–2].

In particular, viral infection represents the main cause of admission and could lead to the need of mechanical ventilation, or extracorporeal oxygenation. Severe bronchiolitis is characterized by increase in airway resistance due to small airway obstruction triggered by inflammation, decrease in lung compliance, and rapid shallow breathing pattern [3–4].

Alveolar collapse and atelectasis are common and lead to lung collapse. In these patients the application of 6–7 cmH$_2$O CPAP delivered by helmet or nasal mask resulted in unloading of respiratory muscles, reduction in respiratory distress, and improvement in gas exchange [5–7].

However, the application of noninvasive respiratory support [NRS] delivered as noninvasive continuous positive airway pressure [nCPAP] or bilevel pressure support often needs PICU or need of high-dependency unit admission. More recently oxygen therapy delivered by high-flow nasal cannula [HFNC] was introduced both in adults and pediatric population [8–11].

Recent studies have reported that HFNC in adults and children improves oxygenation, reduces respiratory drive, and prevents reintubation in high patient risk [12].

HFNC application is easier compared to NRS and often it could be applied in medical ward, whereas NRS use is restricted to the high-dependency units or PICUs. HFNC therapy could result in several clinical benefits by reducing inspiratory effort and work of breathing, increasing end-expiratory volume and CO$_2$ washout for

G. Chidini (✉) · E. Calderini
Pediatric Intensive Care Unit, Fondazione IRCCS Ca Granda Ospedale Maggiore Policlinico, Milan, Italy
e-mail: Giovanna.chidini@policlinico.mi.it

© Springer Nature Switzerland AG 2021
A. Carlucci, S. M. Maggiore (eds.), *High Flow Nasal Cannula*,
https://doi.org/10.1007/978-3-030-42454-1_10

upper airways, and creating a CPAP effect in the upper airways with a CPAP level of 2–3 cmH_2O [13].

This CPAP effect combined with an increase in CO_2 washout and optimal airway humidification could decrease the respiratory work of breathing and improve gas exchange in children [14–15].

The aim of this chapter is to define pediatric ARF and the rationale to apply HFNC and to clarify the mechanism by which HFNC can improve the respiratory mechanics and affect the clinical outcome of children with mild-to-moderate ARF.

10.2 Definitions of Pediatric Acute Respiratory Failure [ARF]

Pediatric respiratory failure consists of several different disease entities, with different pathophysiologies. It is the result of an imbalance between the respiratory muscle power and the respiratory load. ARF in children can be caused by lung [hypoxemic ARF] or respiratory muscle failure [hypercapnic ARF] or by both the conditions. However, although children and adults share a number of physiologic basic respiratory features, small children are prone to develop respiratory failure because of very high chest wall compliance that impedes the neonate's ability to generate adequate tidal volumes and increases the work of breathing [WOB] [16, 17]. The highly compliant chest wall also results in a static functional residual capacity [FRC] that may be decreased to a level at which airway closure, atelectasis, and ventilation/perfusion mismatch occur. The airways of young children have very high flow resistance. Airways are small and gas conductance is low in the peripheral airways, so that a small degree of obstruction due to several causes will result in an unproportional high increase in airway resistance, when compared to adults [18].

Expiratory flows are obstructed due not only to the small dimensions of the airways but also to the altered compliance of the airways and the low FRC generating airway closure during tidal breathing. Apneas are more frequent than in adults and linked to rapid eye movement [REM] sleep, which is more abundant the younger the child is.

Hypoxemic acute respiratory failure is characterized by hypoxemia associated to low or normal carbon dioxide level. With the exception of patients with congenital heart disease and intracardiac right-to-left shunting, the mechanism leading to hypoxemia is ventilation-perfusion mismatch.

Hypoxemic respiratory failure mainly occurs in parenchymal pathologies, such as bacterial and viral pneumonia as well as airway obstruction [i.e., asthma, bronchiolitis] or both [i.e., bronchiolitis, bronchopneumonia, bronchopulmonary dysplasia].

However, if the force generated by the respiratory muscle pump [fatigue or weakness] or central respiratory drive is too low and/or the respiratory load is too high alveolar ventilation may be inadequate, resulting in hypercapnia. It can be "acute" when the unbalance is produced by an acute condition [e.g., acute exacerbation of an asthmatic patients] or defined as "chronic" when the surge is slow during the course of a disease [e.g., neuromuscular disease].

Conventional management of ARF consists of endotracheal intubation with their associated risks such as need for sedation, infections, ventilator-associated pneumonia, and laryngeal-tracheal damage [19, 20]. NRS is an alternative form of respiratory treatment which includes various techniques directed to improve alveolar ventilation, oxygenation, and unloading of respiratory muscles without the need of an endotracheal tube. NRS includes noninvasive continuous positive airway pressure [nCPAP] and noninvasive positive pressure ventilation [nPPV] delivered via an interface [nasal/facial mask or helmet] and ICU or home ventilators [21–23].

Main physiological effects of CPAP are prevention of atelectasis, increase in functional residual capacity reduction in work of breathing, increase in oxygenation, and reduction in left ventricular afterload.

During nPPV the patient's spontaneous inspiratory effort triggers the ventilator to provide a variable flow of gas that increases until airway pressure reaches a selected level. Thus, during each spontaneous inspiration, the patient receives a pressure-supported breath. Differently from nCPAP, nPPV allows a better respiratory system muscle unloading, alveolar recruitment, oxygenation, and carbon dioxide washout improvement.

10.3 Pediatric Physiological Studies

More recently oxygen therapy delivered by high-flow nasal cannula [HFNC] was introduced both in adults and pediatric population.

HFNC is a noninvasive form of respiratory support that can reduce reintubation rates and mortality of patients with acute hypoxemic respiratory failure both in adults and pediatric population. HFNC application is easier compared to NRS and often HFNC as applied in medical ward, whereas NRS use is restricted to the high-dependency units or PICUs. However, the physiologic effects potentially underlying these clinical benefits in children are still largely undefined.

Studies from adult critical care population report the physiological mechanism by which HFNC improves the respiratory function during ARF.

In a prospective randomized physiological controlled study in 15 nonintubated patients with ARF defined by P/F < 300 mmHg, Mauri et al. compared HFNC 40 l/min vs. standard oxygen mask. At the end of each trial, effort of breathing, pressure time product, and change in lung volume were estimated in each group. Results from this study showed that, compared to standard oxygen mask, HFNC improved oxygenation and reduced respiratory rate, esophageal pressure swing, and pressure time product. Moreover, minute ventilation and arterial carbon dioxide tension reduced with an increase in lung volume. Authors found even an increase in dynamic lung compliance and a more homogeneous ventilation distribution. In this population HFNC therapy was associated with several physiological effects such as a reduction in inspiratory effort and an improvement in lung volume and compliance [24].

Flow rate seems to be the principal variable affecting inspiratory effort, lung aeration, and oxygenation, with the maximum effect on inspiratory load and carbon dioxide clearance occurring at relatively low flow rate [30 l/min]. In contrast higher flow rates were associated with a more pronounced increase in oxygenation and reduction in respiratory effort and lung aeration according to a linear correlation model [60 l/min] [25].

Actually, only few neonatal/pediatric studies are published about the physiological effects of HFNC in pediatric ARF.

In a bench study, conducted to quantify the effect of HFNC setting in age-specific lung and airway model, Nielsen et al. found that increasing HFNC flow provided a nonlinear increase in PEEP in a closed-mouth system with maximum tested flows generating 6 cmH_2O in preterm model and 20 cmH_2O in child model. PEEP decreased by 50% in the open-mouth model. The increase in HFNC flow enhanced carbon dioxide washout at a flow of 4 l/min in preterm to 10 l/min in a small child [26].

In a prospective randomized controlled study conducted on HFNC effects on bronchopulmonary dysplasia, 20 infants [mean gestational age 27 weeks, studied at mean postnatal age 30 weeks] were randomized to receive NCPAP or HFNC at day 1, the order being reversed at day 2.

Work of breathing was determined by measuring transdiaphragmatic pressure time product. In this study conducted on infants with evolving or established BPD, no differences were found between the two treatments in terms of work of breathing or oxygenation [27].

In a prospective physiological study conducted on 25 patients [median age 6.5 months, weight 6.4 kg, mainly postoperative children] receiving HFNC, an increasing flow rate was associated with a decreased pressure rate product and esophageal pressure time product [PTP] with the maximum effect seen from 2 to 8 l/min. No side effects were found during the study and no patients required reintubation at 24 h [28].

In a physiological study by Pham et al., electrical diaphragm activity, PRP, esophageal PTP, and change in lung volume were measured during HFNC 2 l/kg in 12 infants with bronchiolitis and 14 cardiac infants. A significant increase in lung volume was found in the bronchiolitis group, associated with a decrease in maximum Edi and PRP during HFNC 2 l/kg whereas a less pronounced effect on diaphragm was found in cardiac patients [29].

In a single-center prospective physiological trial on 21 children less than 3 years old [bronchiolitis and pneumonia], Weiler et al. determined the effects of three different flow rates [0.5, 1.5, and 2 l/kg] on pressure rate product [PRP] with two different HFNC systems.

In this study there was a significant difference in the percent change in PRP from baseline with increasing flow rates for the entire cohort with largest change at 2.0 L/kg/min [21% less]. The optimal HFNC flow rate to reduce the effort of breathing in infants and young children was approximately 1.5–2.0 L/kg/min with more benefit seen in children ≤8 kg [30].

In a recent study comparing HFNC 2 l/kg vs. HFNC 3 l/kg conducted across 16 PICUs and including 244 infants with mild-to-moderate bronchiolitis, Milesi et al. reported a comparable failure rate between groups defined by predetermined criteria in the first 48 hours from admission [38.7% vs. 38.9%, $p = 0.38$]. Worsening comfort was the more common cause of failure in 3 l/kg group. Children in 3 l/kg group had even longer PICU stay [6.4 vs. 5 days, $p = 0.048$]. Intubation rate was not different between groups. No patients had major collateral effects [31].

10.4   Outcome Pediatric Studies

Randomized controlled trials in pediatric subjects are relatively limited. A recent Cochrane review was unable to make any recommendations due to no studies meeting their entry criteria [32].

Nowadays, however few papers are published comparing the physiological effects of HFNC vs. more conventional assistance such as standard oxygen therapy or noninvasive continuous positive airway pressure [nCPAP].

In a multicenter, randomized, controlled trial, conducted by Franklin et al., 1472 infants younger than 12 months with mild-to-moderate bronchiolitis were randomly assigned to receive either high-flow oxygen therapy [high-flow group] or standard oxygen therapy [standard-therapy group]. In this study the primary outcome was escalation of care due to treatment failure defined by predetermined criteria [hypoxemia, tachypnea, worsening in respiratory distress].

In this study the percentage of infants receiving escalation of care was 12% [87 of 739 infants] in the high-flow group, as compared with 23% [167 of 733] in the standard-therapy group [$p < 0.001$]. No significant differences were observed in the duration of hospital stay or the duration of oxygen therapy. Authors concluded that infants with bronchiolitis receiving HFNC outside an ICU had significantly lower rates of escalation of care due to treatment failure than those in the group that received standard oxygen therapy [33].

The first study comparing HFNC vs. nCPAP in terms of outcome was published in 2017 by the French group of Milesi et al. A randomized controlled trials cinducted in five PICUs including 142 infants receiving 7 cmH2O nCPAP vs. 2 l/kg/min HFNC in infants up to 6 months with moderate-to-severe bronchiolitis suggested a relative risk of success 1.63 [95% CI 1.02–2.63] higher with nCPAP. In this study, the superiority analysis showed a risk of success in CPAP group 1.63 [95% CI 1.02–2.63] higher [34].

In a prospective randomized observational study conducted on children aged 2–24 months with ARF, Vitaliti et al. compared CPAP delivered by the pediatric helmet and HFNC therapy [1:1] vs. a control group of patients treated with standard medical treatment. In this study, both HFNC and CPAP were associated with an improvement in oxygenation and respiratory parameters compared with the control group. Helmet CPAP was associated with a more rapid improvement and resolution of respiratory impairment compared to HFNC group [35].

In a recent meta-analysis by Lin et al. including 9 RCT with 2121 included children with mild-to-moderate bronchiolitis, HFNC was found to be safe in the initial treatment; it may have decreased the rate of failure compared to standard oxygen therapy, but it was not associated with an improvement compared to conventional nasal CPAP treatment. An increase in the risk of failure in HFNC group was found compared to nCPAP group. However HFNC was superior to standard oxygen treatment in reducing the risk of failure and hospital length of stay in low- and middle-income countries [36].

In a recent multicenter pilot RCT comparing HFNC vs. nasal CPAP in 254 children with moderate bronchiolitis, Ramnarayan et al. found that more patients were switched from HFNC to nCPAP, thus escalating the treatment, whereas no differences were found between treatment in terms of intubation rate [25.4% of HFNC group vs. 18% in nCPAP group, $p = 0.38$].

On the other side, in an open phase 4 RCT conducted on 202 children with severe bronchiolitis assigned to receive HFNC therapy vs. standard oxygen therapy, HFNC did not reduce time on oxygen compared to standard treatment. Data from this study suggest that HFNC does not affect outcome variables in more severe diseases [37].

In a prospective observational study conducted in a French PICU during two consecutive seasons, the percentage of children treated with HFNC, nCPAP, and bilevel support was analyzed. The main cause of failure among children treated with HFNC was persistent hypercapnia. In this study, arterial carbon dioxide tension was independently associated as a factor for HFNC failure in a multivariate analysis. In this study, authors found that HFNC can potentially decrease the use of nCPAP, the limiting factor being the increase in arterial carbon dioxide level [38].

10.5 Conclusions

Nowadays, several reviews and meta-analysis suggest that HFNC is safe as an initial respiratory management in children with mild-to-moderate ARF due to infectious diseases. In this population HFNC therapy could result in several clinical benefits by reducing inspiratory effort and work of breathing, increasing end-expiratory volume and CO_2 washout for upper airways, and creating a positive pressure effect in the upper airways with a level of 2–3 cmH_2O. These effects combined with an optimal airway humidification could decrease the respiratory work of breathing and improve gas exchange. However, studies comparing HFNC therapy vs. more conventional approach with nCPAP showed a noninferiority effect of nCPAP, showing that nCPAP could be associated with a more favorable outcome in children with more severe disease. Elevated values of arterial carbon dioxide and high indexes of respiratory work of breathing [such as PRP and esophageal PTP] seem to be associated with HFNC failure and the need of escalating the respiratory support. Initial setting with a flow rate of 2 l/kg seems to be associated with the greater reduction in respiratory effort in acutely ill infants, with a more favorable outcome compared with standard oxygen therapy.

On the other side, further randomized controlled studies are needed to compare the efficacy of HFNC to that of more conventional noninvasive support such as nCPAP and bilevel ventilation.

References

1. Balfour Lynn RE, Marsh G, Gorayi D, et al. Non-invasive ventilation for children with acute respiratory failure in the developing world: literature review and implementation example. Paediatr Respir Rev. 2014;15:181–7.
2. Murthy S, Kissoon N. Management of severe viral infections in the pediatric intensive care unit. J Pediatr Intens Care. 2014;3:205–16.
3. Ganu SS, Gautam A, Wilkins B, et al. Increase in use of non-invasive ventilation for infants with severe bronchiolitis is associated with decline in intubation rates over a decade. Intensive Care Med. 2012;38:1177–83.
4. Essouri S, Laurent M, Chevret L, et al. Improved clinical and economic outcomes in severe bronchiolitis with pre-emptive nCPAP ventilatory strategy. Intensive Care Med. 2014;40(1):84–91.
5. Milesi C. Matecki S, Jaber S, Thibaut M, Jaquot A, Pidoux O et al. 6 cmH$_2$O Cntinuous Positive Airway Pressure versus conventional oxygen therapy in severe viral bronchiolitis: a randomized trial. Pediatri Pulmonol. 2013;48:45–51.
6. Chidini G, Piastra M, Marchesi T, De Luca D, Napolitano L, Salvo I, Wolfler A, Pelosi P, Damasco M, Conti G, Calderini E. Continuous positive airway pressure with helmet versus mask in infants with bronchiolitis: an RCT. Pediatrics. 2015;135(4):e86875. https://doi.org/10.1542/peds.2014-1142. Epub 2015 Mar 15
7. Chidini G, Calderini E, Pelosi P. Treatment of acute hypoxemic respiratory failure with continuous positive airway pressure delivered by a new pediatric helmet in comparison with a standard full face mask: a prospective pilot study. Pediatr Crit Care Med. 2010;11:502–8.
8. Papazian L, Corley A, Hess D, Fraser JF, Frat JP, Guitton C, Jaber S, Maggiore SM, Nava S, Rello J, Ricard JD, Stephan F, Trisolini R, Azoulay E. Use of high-flow nasal cannula oxygenation in ICU adults: a narrative review. Intensive Care Med. 2016;42:1336–49.
9. Nishimura M. High-flow nasal cannula oxygen therapy in adults: physiological benefits, indication, clinical benefits, and adverse effects. Respir Care. 2016;61(4):529–41.
10. Maggiore SM, Idone FA, Vaschetto R, Festa R, Cataldo A, Antonicelli F, Montini L, De Gaetano A, Navalesi P, Antonelli M. Nasal high flow versus Venturi mask oxygen therapy after extubation. Effects on oxygenation, comfort, and clinical outcome. Am J Respir Crit Care Med. 2014;190:282–8.
11. Frat JP, Thille AW, Mercat A, Girault C, Ragot S, Perbet S, Prat G, Boulain T, Morawiec E, Cottereau A, Devaquet J, Nseir S, Razazi K, Mira JP, Argaud L, Chakarian JC, Ricard JD, Wittebole X, Chevalier S, Herbland A, Fartoukh M, Constantin JM, Tonnelier JM, Pierrot M, Mathonnet A, Béduneau G, Delétage-Métreau C, Richard JC, Brochard L, Robert R. High-flow oxygen through nasal cannula: FLORALI study group; REVA network. New Eng J Med. 2015;372:2185–96.
12. Shibler A, Pham TMT, Dunster KR, Foster K, et al. Reduced intubation rate for infants after introduction of high flow nasal prong oxygen delivery. Intensive Care Med. 2011;37:847–52.
13. Mauri T, Alban L, Turrini C, Cambiaghi B, Carlesso E, Taccone P, Bottino N, Lissoni A, Spadaro S, Volta CA, Gattinoni L, Pesenti A, Grasselli G. Optimum support by high flow nasal cannula in acute hypoxemic respiratory failure: effects of increasing flow rates. Intensive Care Med. https://doi.org/10.1007/s00134-017-4890.
14. Lee JH, Rehder KJ, Williford L, Cheifetz IM, Turner DA. Use of high flow nasal cannula in critically ill infants, children, and adults: a critical review of the literature. Intensive Care Med. 2013;39:247–57.
15. Pham TM, O'Malley L, Mayfield S, Martin S, Schibler A. The effect of high flow nasal cannula therapy on the work of breathing in infants with bronchiolitis. Pediatr Pulmonol. 2015;50:713–20.
16. Hagan R, Bryan AC, Bryan MH, Gulston G. Neonatal chest wall afferents and regulation of respiration. J Appl Physiol. 1977;42:362–7.
17. Guslits BG, Gaston SE, Bryan MH, England SJ, Bryan AC. Diaphragmatic work of breathing in premature human infants. J Appl Physiol. 1987;62:1410–5.

18. Bryan AC, Wohl MEB. Respiratory mechanics in children. Handbook of physiology. Section 3: the respiratory system, volume III: mechanics of breathing, part 1. Bethesda: American Physiological Society, Williams & Wilkins; 1986. p. 179–91.

19. Orlowski JP, Ellis NG, Amin NP, et al. Complications of airway intrusion in 100 consecutive cases in a pediatric ICU. Crit Care Med. 1980;8:324–31.

20. Craven DE, Kunches LM, Kilinsky V, et al. Risk factors for pneumonia and fatality in patients receiving continuous mechanical ventilation. Am Rev Respir Dis. 1986;133:792–6.

21. Essouri S, Nicot F, Clement A, et al. Noninvasive positive pressure ventilation in infants with upper airway obstruction: comparison of continuous and bilevel positive pressure. Intensive Care Med. 2005;31:574–80.

22. Morley CJ, Davis PG, Doyle LW, for the COIN Trial Investigators, et al. Nasal CPAP or intubation at birth for very preterm infants. N Engl J Med. 2008;358:700–8.

23. Gregoretti C, Pelosi P, Chidini G, Bignamini E, Calderini E. Noninvasive ventilation in pediatric intensive care. Noninvasive ventilation in pediatric intensive care. Minerva Pediatr. 2010;62:437–58.

24. Mauri T, Turrini C, Eronia N, Grasselli G, Volta CA, Bellani G, Pesenti A. Physiologic effects of high-flow nasal cannula in acute hypoxemic respiratory failure. Am J Respir Crit Care Med. 2017;195:1207–15.

25. Mauri T, Alban L, Turrini C, Cambiaghi B, Carlesso E, Taccone P, Bottino N, Lissoni A, Spadaro S, Volta CA, Gattinoni L, Pesenti A, Grasselli G. Optimum support by high-flow nasal cannula in acute hypoxemic respiratory failure: effects of increasing flow rates. Intensive Care Med. 2017;43:1453–63.

26. Nielsen KR, Ellington EL, Gray AJ, Stanberry LI, Smith LS, DiBlasi RM. Effect of high-flow nasal cannula on expiratory pressure and ventilation in infant, pediatric, and adult models. Respir Care. Paper in Press. Published on October 24, 2017 as. https://doi.org/10.4187/respcare.05728.

27. Shetty Sm Hickey A, Rafferty GF, Peacock JL, Grrenough A. Work of breathing during CPAP and heated humidified high-flow nasal cannula. Arch Dis Child Fetal Neonatal Ed. 2016:F1–4.

28. Rubin S, Guman A, Deakers T, Khemani R, Ross P, Newth CJ. Effort of breathing in children receiving high flow nasal cannulas. Pediatr Critic Care Med. 2014;15:1–6.

29. Pham TM, O'Malley L, Mayfield S, Martin S, Schibler A. The effect of high flow nasal cannula therapy on the work of breathing in infants with bronchiolitis. Pediatr Pulmonol. 2015;50:713–20.

30. Weiler T, Kamerkar A, Hotz J, Ross PA, Newth CJ, Khemani RG. The relationship between high flow nasal cannula flow rate and effort of breathing in children. J Pediatr. 2017;189:66–71.

31. Milesi C, Pierre AF, Deho A, Liets JM, et al. Multicenter randomized controlled trial of a 3-L/kg/min versus 2-L/kg/min high-flow nasal cannula flow rate in young infants with severe viral bronchiolitis [TRAMONTANE 2]. Intensive Care Med. 2018;44:1870–8.

32. Mayfield S, Jauncey-Cooke J, Hough JL, Schibler A, Gibbons K, Bogossian F. High-flow nasal cannula therapy for respiratory support in children. Cochrane Database Syst Rev. 2014;3:CD009850.

33. Franklin D, Babl FE, Schlapbach LJ, Oakley E, Craig S, Neutze J, Furyk J, Fraser JF, Jones M, Whitty JA, Dalziel SR, Schibler. A randomized trial of high-flow therapy in infants with bronchiolitis. N Engl J Med. 2018;378:1121–31.

34. Milési C, Essouri S, Pouyau R, Liet J-M, Afanetti M, Portefaix A, et al. High flow nasal cannula [HFNC] versus nasal continuous positive airway pressure [nCPAP] for the initial respiratory management of acute viral bronchiolitis in young infants: a multicenter randomized controlled trial [TRAMONTANE study]. Intensive Care Med. 2017;43:209–16.

35. Vitaliti G, Vitaliti MG, Finocchiaro MC, Di Stefano VA, et al. Randomized comparison of helmet CPAP versus high-flow nasal cannula oxygen in Pediatric respiratory distress. Respir Care. 2017;62:1036–42.

36. Lin J, Zhang Y, Xiong L, Liu S, Gong C, Dai J. High-flow nasal cannula therapy for children with bronchiolitis: a systematic review and meta-analysis. Arch Dis Child. 2019:1–13.

37. Kepreotes E, Whitehead B, Attia J, Oldmeadow C, Collison A, Searles A, et al. High-flow warm humidified oxygen versus standard low-flow nasal cannula oxygen for moderate bronchiolitis [HFWHO RCT]: an open, phase 4, randomised controlled trial. Lancet. 2017;389:930–9.
38. Guillot C, Le Reun C, Behal H, Labreuche J, Recher M, Duhamel A, Leteurtre S. First line treatment using high flow nasal cannula for children with severe bronchiolitis: applicability and risk factors for failure. Archives de Pediatrie. 2018;25:213–8.

Future Perspectives

11

Oriol Roca and Marina García-De-Acilu

11.1 Introduction

Since the first description of the use of high-flow nasal cannula (HFNC) supportive therapy in adult patients in 2010 [1], and especially since the publication of the FLORALI trial [2], its use in adult patients has spread rapidly.

After an initial burst of enthusiasm, however, the first negative trials appeared and the optimism began to cool. So, even though it is quite clear that HFNC is not harmful and offers several physiological benefits [3, 4], a number of questions regarding its use remain unanswered.

In this chapter, we review the future prospects of HFNC and suggest possible lines of research that focus on the issues that remain unresolved at present: namely, personalized flow titration, usefulness of the treatment in specific clinical situations and respiratory failure etiologies, and early identification of patients who will fail after HFNC.

11.2 How Should HFNC be Used?

HFNC appears to be a straightforward, easy-to-apply procedure, and there are no clear recommendations regarding its use. What is clear is that current practices are physiologically based. The effects of HFNC are flow dependent [3, 4] and the

O. Roca (✉)
Intensive Care Department, Vall d'Hebron University Hospital, Vall d'Hebron Research Institute, Universitat Autònoma de Barcelona, Barcelona, Spain

Ciber Enfermedades Respiratorias (Ciberes), Instituto de Salud Carlos III, Madrid, Spain
e-mail: oroca@vhebron.net

M. García-De-Acilu
Intensive Care Department, Vall d'Hebron University Hospital, Vall d'Hebron Research Institute, Universitat Autònoma de Barcelona, Barcelona, Spain

© Springer Nature Switzerland AG 2021
A. Carlucci, S. M. Maggiore (eds.), *High Flow Nasal Cannula*,
https://doi.org/10.1007/978-3-030-42454-1_11

treatment has traditionally been used in acute hypoxemic respiratory failure (AHRF) at the maximum tolerated flow. The same approach has also been used to prevent respiratory failure after extubation [5]. However, the maximum flow tolerated in this latter situation is normally lower than that tolerated by a patient with AHRF and high inspiratory flow demand. Thus, even though the flow titration approach is the same, the final flow rate used may change according to tolerability, which is highly influenced by the clinical situation of each patient.

Compared to low-flow conventional oxygen, HFNC in patients with AHRF reduces the inspiratory effort, respiratory rate (RR), and minute ventilation without changes in $PaCO_2$, consistent with dead-space washout, and improves oxygenation [4]. It also improves dynamic compliance and the homogeneity of the distribution of inhaled gas, and increases transpulmonary pressures while reducing transpulmonary driving pressure. Moreover, during HFNC use and with increasing flow rates there is a linear decrease in RR, an increase in end-expiratory lung volume (EELV), and improvements in lung mechanics and oxygenation [3]. In contrast, most gains in terms of minute ventilation are already obtained at 30 Lpm. Therefore, personalized bedside titration of the flow rate may be desirable in order to achieve maximum clinical benefit during HFNC therapy.

Interestingly, tidal volume (V_t) is not affected by increases in flow rate up to 60 Lpm. Moreover, as we noted above, RR, EELV, lung mechanics, and oxygenation improve linearly up to 60 Lpm; therefore, the use of flows higher than 60 Lpm may be associated with greater improvements, as it is in healthy volunteers [6], and therefore, may be beneficial in some patients. In fact, it needs to be confirmed whether flows >60 Lpm can be used for a short period of time in patients who continue to show signs of respiratory distress at 60 Lpm, or as an initial therapy in patients with severe AHRF.

Another point that should be analyzed in longer periods of HFNC is how flow and temperature affect comfort and treatment tolerability. This issue has already been tested in a study period of 20 minutes, when, for any given flow rate, a lower temperature (31 °C) resulted in better patient comfort [7]. As expected, better comfort was observed in more severe patients with $F_iO_2 \geq 0.45$ with higher flow rates (60 Lpm). Thus, although the ideal temperature of gas delivery may be 37 °C, the issue of whether lowering the temperature improves comfort in long-term HFNC use should be assessed. Likewise, flow titration should be guided by patient comfort, as patient experience varies widely.

As in the case of flow titration, little is known about weaning from HFNC. There is no clear recommendation at present; making an analogy with standard practice in patients who are mechanically ventilated with F_iO_2 and PEEP, it seems reasonable to start by decreasing F_iO_2 and then reducing the flow. The other point that should also be clarified is when patients can be transitioned to standard O_2 therapy. Should the flow be reduced below 30 Lpm, or maybe below 20Lpm, before performing the conventional oxygen trial? All these strategies need to be tested in randomized trials.

11.3 Specific AHRF Etiologies

The effectiveness of HFNC in specific AHRF etiologies should also be examined. The publication of the FLORALI trial, which included patients with AHRF of different etiologies, was met with great enthusiasm—so much so that HFNC may now be overused. However, we clearly need to define the patients in whom HFNC is useful and those in which it is not. For example, the more recently published HIGH trial found that HFNC was not superior to conventional oxygen in a large population of immunocompromised patients [8]. Nonetheless, one should bear in mind that very often it is extremely difficult to demonstrate any benefit in outcomes in critically ill patients; indeed, the outcomes of immunocompromised patients may be strongly influenced by their premorbid condition when the respiratory failure occurs. Moreover, one might think that HFNC needs to demonstrate superiority to conventional oxygen in terms of outcomes, but, if it proves to be more comfortable for the patients, perhaps it only needs to demonstrate non-inferiority. In fact, the same reasoning was used in some trials comparing HFNC with NIV [9].

Evidence in many specific patient populations is still lacking. Although noninvasive ventilation is the gold standard therapy for COPD exacerbation [10], evidence of HFNC use in these patients is steadily increasing. It has been shown that HFNC leads to a flow-dependent reduction in pCO_2, most likely achieved by a washout of the respiratory tract and a functional reduction in dead space [11]. These results suggest that HFNC enhances the effectiveness of breathing in patients with COPD, reducing pCO_2 and work of breathing. Compared to NIV, HFNC is easier to apply, is more comfortable for patients and more convenient for medical staff, has fewer undesirable effects, and is probably cheaper. For this reason, and in view of the encouraging physiological benefits, the first randomized trials comparing HFNC versus NIV (ClinicalTrials.gov ID: NCT03033251 and NCT03014869) or versus conventional oxygen between NIV sessions (ClinicalTrials.gov ID: NCT03406572) in COPD exacerbation are currently underway.

A similar case is acute cardiogenic pulmonary edema, in which NIV or CPAP is considered the standard of use [10]. However, HFNC is more comfortable and easier to use and it may induce similar cardiovascular benefits to NIV or CPAP [12]. To date, only one randomized trial has been performed to compare HFNC with conventional oxygen [13]. The primary outcome was respiratory rate 60 minutes postintervention, which showed a reduction of 3.3 (95% CI 1.9–4.6) bpm. Only 128 patients were included, and no differences in important outcomes such as intubation rates or mortality were found. Therefore, larger randomized trials specifically designed to detect differences in such important outcomes in this specific population are desirable.

11.4   Predictors of HFNC Failure

The benefits of HFNC should be carefully balanced against its risks. One important concern with HFNC use is that, by masking the signs of respiratory distress, it may delay an inevitable intubation and thus worsen patient outcomes [14, 15]. Thus, the search for early predictors of HFNC failure is a field of special interest. The first studies only reported the variables associated with a higher risk of HFNC failure: the absence of oxygenation improvement [16–18], the persistence of high RR or thoracoabdominal asynchrony [17], the need for vasopressors [16, 18, 19], higher disease severity [20], higher baseline SOFA score [21, 22], and the extent of pleural effusion [21]. However, none of these variables has been tested prospectively to predict HFNC outcome, and only two studies have examined their diagnostic accuracy: a secondary analysis of the FLORALI study which showed that higher heart rate was independently associated with intubation in HFNC patients with an area under the ROC curve (AUROC) of 0.657 for predicting intubation [23], and an assessment of the ROX index, defined as the ratio of SpO_2/F_IO_2 to RR, which outperformed either variable alone in terms of diagnostic accuracy with an AUROC of 0.74 [24]. Patients with a ROX index ≥ 4.88 after 12 hours of HFNC therapy were less likely to be intubated (HR 0.27 [95% CI 0.12–0.62]), even after adjusting for potential covariates. Moreover, dynamic changes of the ROX index may also be useful. Among patients who were still on HFNC after 18 h, the median change in the ROX index between 12 h and 18 h was significantly higher in patients who did not require intubation.

More recently, the utility of the ROX index was prospectively validated in a multicenter study [25]. The results confirmed that a ROX index ≥ 4.88 measured at 2, 6, or 12 h was a determinant of HFNC success, even after adjusting for potential confounding variables. By contrast, ROX indexes below 2.85, 3.47, and 3.85 at 2, 6, and 12 h after HFNC initiation allowed identification of HFNC failure with a very high specificity. Again, dynamic changes in the ROX were also important and patients who failed presented a smaller increase in ROX index values from 2 to 12 and 6 to 12 h compared to those patients who succeeded. These differences in the ROX index were associated with the risk of HFNC failure after adjusting for the value of the ROX index at the beginning of the period analyzed. It should also be noted that patients intubated within the first 12 hours of treatment did not present any excess of mortality. We therefore suggest that the ROX index should be monitored over time, focusing especially on the 12th hour onwards: if the ROX is ≥ 4.88, the patient has a high chance of success, but if it is <3.85, the risk of failure is high and intubation should be considered. Obviously there is a gray zone between 3.85 and 4.88, where dynamic changes in the ROX may be useful. If a patient is in the gray zone at 12 h, the ROX could be repeated 1 or 2 h later: (1) if the score has risen, the likelihood of success is greater; (2) if it has fallen, then intubation is more likely to be required; and (3) if the score is unchanged then reassessment should be performed after one or two more hours. However, a strategy of this kind will obviously require a prospective evaluation, which is currently ongoing in a randomized trial (ClinicalTrials.gov ID: NCT04707729).

Finally, it should be noted that the value of the ROX index might be influenced by the flow rate used, as in the case of oxygenation and PEEP in patients with mechanical ventilation [26]. This increase in the ROX after raising the flow may be the result of a recruitment effect and/or decreasing the dead space or work of breathing; therefore, one might hypothesize that, if this increase does not materialize, the patient would not succeed on HFNC and would need to be intubated. Thus, standardizing the measurement of the ROX to a specific level of flow could be of interest. Similarly, the value of the ROX as well as its diagnostic accuracy may be influenced by the use of different intubation criteria. Indeed, the use of the ROX index should be tested in a randomized controlled trial comparing traditional intubation criteria alone to these traditional criteria with the addition of the use of ROX.

Another important area of research with regard to predicting HFNC failure is patient phenotyping. Different ARDS phenotypes have been associated with different outcomes and treatment responses [27]. As in the case of the hyperinflammatory ARDS phenotype, higher plasma concentrations of interleukin (IL) 8 within 24 h of ARF onset were observed in patients who failed on HFNC in a relatively small cohort of patients with hypoxemic ARF with bilateral infiltrates [28]. Furthermore, levels of IL-8 ≥ 67.16 pg/mL independently predict the need for mechanical ventilation in patients treated with HFNC after adjusting for severity. These results suggest that defining distinct subgroups or phenotypes of HFNC patients may be important for the design of future randomized clinical trials; it may help us to understand the pathophysiology of treatment failure and to identify patients who are at a higher risk of failure at an early stage.

11.5 HFNC in Sepsis

Although the need for vasopressors has been an exclusion criterion in some randomized trials using HFNC [2], it should be noted that many patients treated with HFNC have sepsis. For its part, fluid overload has traditionally been considered as a cause of intubation in patients with respiratory failure. Taking these two concepts together, it makes sense to investigate predictors of fluid responsiveness that may improve fluid management and as a result lower intubation rates in these patients.

Moreover, in view of the physiological benefits described [3, 4], it is likely that HFNC may prevent patient self-inflicted lung injury [29] in non-hypoxemic patients at risk of developing this condition. Hopefully, the results of the OPTISEPSIS study (NCT03334227) will shed further light on this issue.

11.6 Conclusions

High-flow nasal cannula has changed the paradigm of management of patients with respiratory failure and provides substantial physiological benefits. However, several questions regarding this treatment remain unanswered; future research should focus on how it should be used, which patients benefit the most, and how to achieve prompt identification of patients who will fail on HFNC at an early stage, so as not to delay intubation in cases in which it is necessary.

Acknowledgements and Conflicts of Interest OR discloses research grant from Hamilton Medical and speaker fees from Hamilton Medical, Ambu and Aerogen Ltd, and non-financial research support from Timpel and Masimo Corporation. His insitution received fees for consultancy from Hamilton Medical. MG has no conflicts of interest to disclose.

References

1. Roca O, Riera J, Torres F, Masclans JR. High-flow oxygen therapy in acute respiratory failure. Respir Care. 2010;55:408–13.
2. Frat JP, Thille AW, Mercat A, Girault C, Ragot S, Perbet S, Prat G, Boulain T, Morawiec E, Cottereau A, Devaquet J, Nseir S, Razazi K, Mira JP, Argaud L, Chakarian JC, Ricard JD, Wittebole X, Chevalier S, Herbland A, Fartoukh M, Constantin JM, Tonnelier JM, Pierrot M, Mathonnet A, Beduneau G, Deletage-Metreau C, Richard JC, Brochard L, Robert R, Group FS, Network R. High-flow oxygen through nasal cannula in acute hypoxemic respiratory failure. N Engl J Med. 2015;372:2185–96.
3. Mauri T, Alban L, Turrini C, Cambiaghi B, Carlesso E, Taccone P, Bottino N, Lissoni A, Spadaro S, Volta CA, Gattinoni L, Pesenti A, Grasselli G. Optimum support by high-flow nasal cannula in acute hypoxemic respiratory failure: effects of increasing flow rates. Intensive Care Med. 2017;43:1453–63.
4. Mauri T, Turrini C, Eronia N, Grasselli G, Volta CA, Bellani G, Pesenti A. Physiologic effects of high-flow nasal cannula in acute hypoxemic respiratory failure. Am J Respir Crit Care Med. 2017;195:1207–15.
5. Hernandez G, Vaquero C, Gonzalez P, Subira C, Frutos-Vivar F, Rialp G, Laborda C, Colinas L, Cuena R, Fernandez R. Effect of postextubation high-flow nasal cannula vs conventional oxygen therapy on reintubation in low-risk patients: a randomized clinical trial. JAMA. 2016;315:1354–61.
6. Parke RL, Bloch A, McGuinness SP. Effect of very-high-flow nasal therapy on airway pressure and end-expiratory lung impedance in healthy volunteers. Respir Care. 2015;60:1397–403.
7. Mauri T, Galazzi A, Binda F, Masciopinto L, Corcione N, Carlesso E, Lazzeri M, Spinelli E, Tubiolo D, Volta CA, Adamini I, Pesenti A, Grasselli G. Impact of flow and temperature on patient comfort during respiratory support by high-flow nasal cannula. Crit Care. 2018;22:120.
8. Azoulay E, Lemiale V, Mokart D, Nseir S, Argaud L, Pene F, Kontar L, Bruneel F, Klouche K, Barbier F, Reignier J, Berrahil-Meksen L, Louis G, Constantin JM, Mayaux J, Wallet F, Kouatchet A, Peigne V, Theodose I, Perez P, Girault C, Jaber S, Oziel J, Nyunga M, Terzi N, Bouadma L, Lebert C, Lautrette A, Bige N, Raphalen JH, Papazian L, Darmon M, Chevret S, Demoule A. Effect of high-flow nasal oxygen vs. standard oxygen on 28-day mortality in immunocompromised patients with acute respiratory failure: the HIGH randomized clinical trial. JAMA. 2018;320:2099.
9. Hernandez G, Vaquero C, Colinas L, Cuena R, Gonzalez P, Canabal A, Sanchez S, Rodriguez ML, Villasclaras A, Fernandez R. Effect of Postextubation high-flow nasal cannula vs. noninvasive ventilation on reintubation and Postextubation respiratory failure in high-risk patients: a randomized clinical trial. JAMA. 2016;316:1565–74.
10. Rochwerg B, Brochard L, Elliott MW, Hess D, Hill NS, Nava S, Navalesi PMOTSC, Antonelli M, Brozek J, Conti G, Ferrer M, Guntupalli K, Jaber S, Keenan S, Mancebo J, Mehta S, Raoof SMOTTF. Official ERS/ATS clinical practice guidelines: noninvasive ventilation for acute respiratory failure. Eur Respir J. 2017;50:1602426.

11. Braunlich J, Kohler M, Wirtz H. Nasal highflow improves ventilation in patients with COPD. Int J Chron Obstruct Pulmon Dis. 2016;11:1077–85.
12. Roca O, Perez-Teran P, Masclans JR, Perez L, Galve E, Evangelista A, Rello J. Patients with New York Heart Association class III heart failure may benefit with high flow nasal cannula supportive therapy: high flow nasal cannula in heart failure. J Crit Care. 2013;28:741–6.
13. Makdee O, Monsomboon A, Surabenjawong U, Praphruetkit N, Chaisirin W, Chakorn T, Permpikul C, Thiravit P, Nakornchai T. High-flow nasal cannula versus conventional oxygen therapy in emergency department patients with cardiogenic pulmonary edema: a randomized controlled trial. Ann Emerg Med. 2017;70:465–72.e462
14. Kang BJ, Koh Y, Lim CM, Huh JW, Baek S, Han M, Seo HS, Suh HJ, Seo GJ, Kim EY, Hong SB. Failure of high-flow nasal cannula therapy may delay intubation and increase mortality. Intensive Care Med. 2015;41:623–32.
15. Carrillo A, Gonzalez-Diaz G, Ferrer M, Martinez-Quintana ME, Lopez-Martinez A, Llamas N, Alcazar M, Torres A. Non-invasive ventilation in community-acquired pneumonia and severe acute respiratory failure. Intensive Care Med. 2012;38:458–66.
16. Rello J, Perez M, Roca O, Poulakou G, Souto J, Laborda C, Balcells J, Serra J, Masclans JR. High-flow nasal therapy in adults with severe acute respiratory infection: a cohort study in patients with 2009 influenza a/H1N1v. J Crit Care. 2012;27:434–9.
17. Sztrymf B, Messika J, Bertrand F, Hurel D, Leon R, Dreyfuss D, Ricard JD. Beneficial effects of humidified high flow nasal oxygen in critical care patients: a prospective pilot study. Intensive Care Med. 2011;37:1780–6.
18. Hyun Cho W, Ju Yeo H, Hoon Yoon S, Lee S, SooJeon D, Seong Kim Y, Uk Kim K, Lee K, Kyung Park H, Ki LM. High-flow nasal cannula therapy for acute hypoxemic respiratory failure in adults: a retrospective analysis. Intern Med (Tokyo, Japan). 2015;54:2307–13.
19. Roca O, de Acilu MG, Caralt B, Sacanell J, Masclans JR. Humidified high flow nasal cannula supportive therapy improves outcomes in lung transplant recipients readmitted to the intensive care unit because of acute respiratory failure. Transplantation. 2015;99:1092–8.
20. Messika J, Ben Ahmed K, Gaudry S, Miguel-Montanes R, Rafat C, Sztrymf B, Dreyfuss D, Ricard JD. Use of high-flow nasal cannula oxygen therapy in subjects with ARDS: a 1-year observational study. Respir Care. 2015;60:162–9.
21. Koga Y, Kaneda K, Mizuguchi I, Nakahara T, Miyauchi T, Fujita M, Kawamura Y, Oda Y, Tsuruta R. Extent of pleural effusion on chest radiograph is associated with failure of high-flow nasal cannula oxygen therapy. J Crit Care. 2016;32:165–9.
22. Kim WY, Sung H, Hong SB, Lim CM, Koh Y, Huh JW. Predictors of high flow nasal cannula failure in immunocompromised patients with acute respiratory failure due to non-HIV pneumocystis pneumonia. J Thorac Dis. 2017;9:3013–22.
23. Frat JP, Ragot S, Coudroy R, Constantin JM, Girault C, Prat G, Boulain T, Demoule A, Ricard JD, Razazi K, Lascarrou JB, Devaquet J, Mira JP, Argaud L, Chakarian JC, Fartoukh M, Nseir S, Mercat A, Brochard L, Robert R, Thille AW. Predictors of intubation in patients with acute hypoxemic respiratory failure treated with a noninvasive oxygenation strategy. Crit Care Med. 2018;46:208–15.
24. Roca O, Messika J, Caralt B, Garcia-de-Acilu M, Sztrymf B, Ricard JD, Masclans JR. Predicting success of high-flow nasal cannula in pneumonia patients with hypoxemic respiratory failure: the utility of the ROX index. J Crit Care. 2016;35:200–5.
25. Roca O, Caralt B, Messika J, Samper M, Sztrymf B, Hernandez G, Garcia-de-Acilu M, Frat JP, Masclans JR, Ricard JD. An index combining respiratory rate and oxygenation to predict outcome of nasal high flow therapy. Am J Respir Crit Care Med. 2018;199:1368.
26. Carlesso E, Mauri T, Spinelli E, Galazzi A, Binda F, Tortolani D, Turrini C, Alban L, Lazzeri M, Abbruzzese C, Tagliabue P, Spadaro S, Grasselli G, Roca O, Pesenti A. Effects of set flow rate on the ROX index in acute hypoxemic respiratory failure patients undergoing high flow therapy. Intensive Care Med Exp. 2018;6(Suppl 2):222–3.

27. Sinha P, Calfee CS. Phenotypes in acute respiratory distress syndrome: moving towards precision medicine. Curr Opin Crit Care. 2019;25:12–20.
28. Garcia-de-Acilu M, Marin-Corral J, Vazquez A, Ruano L, Magret M, Ferrer R, Masclans JR, Roca O. Hypoxemic patients with bilateral infiltrates treated with high-flow nasal cannula present a similar pattern of biomarkers of inflammation and injury to acute respiratory distress syndrome patients. Crit Care Med. 2017;45:1845–53.
29. Brochard L, Slutsky A, Pesenti A. Mechanical ventilation to minimize progression of lung injury in acute respiratory failure. Am J Respir Crit Care Med. 2017;195:438–42.